OXFORD MEDICAL PUBLICATIONS

Current paediatric cardiology

Current paediatric cardiology

ELLIOT A. SHINEBOURNE
M.D., F.R.C.P.
Consultant Paediatric Cardiologist
Brompton Hospital, London and
Senior Lecturer,
Cardiothoracic Institute, University of London

AND

ROBERT H. ANDERSON
B.Sc., M.D., M.R.C.Path.
Joseph Levy Reader in Paediatric Cardiac Morphology,
Cardiothoracic Institute, University of London and
Honorary Consultant
Brompton Hospital, London

WITH THE COLLABORATION OF
M. De Swiet, A. M. El Seed, K. Fox, O. D. H. Jones,
D. Krikler, J. C. R. Lincoln, M. L. Rigby, T. R. Traill,
and J. R. Zuberbuhler.

OXFORD UNIVERSITY PRESS

Oxford   New York   Toronto

1980

Oxford University Press, Walton Street, Oxford OX2 6DP

OXFORD LONDON GLASGOW
NEW YORK TORONTO MELBOURNE WELLINGTON
KUALA LUMPUR SINGAPORE JAKARTA HONG KONG TOKYO
DELHI BOMBAY CALCUTTA MADRAS KARACHI
IBADAN NAIROBI DAR ES SALAAM CAPE TOWN

British Library Cataloguing in Publication Data

Shinebourne, Elliot A
   Current paediatric cardiology.—(Oxford
   medical publications).
   1. Pediatric cardiology
   I. Title II. Anderson, Robert H
   III. Series
   618.9′21′2   RJ421   79–41184
   ISBN 0–19–261141–0

Set, printed and bound in Great Britain by
Fakenham Press Limited,
Fakenham, Norfolk

Preface

This book has its seed in the section on paediatric cardiology written for the twelfth edition of *Price's Textbook of the practice of medicine*. We felt at that time, and continue to feel now, perhaps from a biased viewpoint, that there is a need for a simple account of paediatric cardiology suitable for general cardiologists and paediatricians, paediatric cardiologists in training, senior medical students, and workers in ancillary fields. This book represents our attempt to provide such an account while at the same time incorporating the anatomical and physiological basis of the subject. It has undergone considerable change from its conception in '*Price*'. This at first related to the need to consider more fully such important topics as differential diagnosis and echocardiography and also to provide accounts of topics such as rheumatic fever, arrhythmias, infective endocarditis, and risk factors, which were covered by other authors in the Textbook of Medicine. When we had asked our colleagues, Bob Zuberbuhler, Tom Traill, Kim Fox, Dennis Krikler, Abdulmoneim El Seed, and Michael de Swiet to assist in the preparation of these chapters, it became evident that many of our other sections were thus unbalanced. These were therefore expanded to varying degrees, and we drew on the assistance of our surgical colleague, Christopher Lincoln, to add the sections on surgical treatment. We hope the resultant volume will provide a simple and brief introduction to current concepts in paediatric cardiology. If it does not, the fault is entirely ours.

ELLIOT A. SHINEBOURNE
ROBERT H. ANDERSON
LONDON, 1979

Acknowledgements

Clearly it would have been impossible to write this book without the assistance, freely given, of our friends and colleagues from the Brompton Hospital and other institutions in London and elsewhere. In particular we are indebted to our contributors, Dr. J. R. Zuberbuhler of Pittsburgh Children's Hospital; Dr. T. R. Traill of Brompton Hospital; Drs K. Fox and D. Krikler of Hammersmith Hospital, London; Dr. Abdulmoneim El Seed of Khartoum University, Sudan; Dr. Michael de Swiet of the Cardiothoracic Institute, London; and Mr. Christopher Lincoln of Brompton Hospital for responding so promptly to our request for chapters and for acceding with minimal dissent to editorial licence. We would also like to thank Professor Fergus Macartney and Drs Michael Tynan, Anton Becker, James L. Wilkinson, and Manuel Quero-Jimenez who have been privy to the formulation of many of the concepts expressed herein. The artwork was provided with consummate skill and customary speed by Siew Yen Ho, and we thank her for this continuing service. Much of the work itself would not have been possible without continuing help and support from the British Heart Foundation and the Joseph Levy Foundation. It is a pleasure to record the willing cooperation provided by our publishers, particularly Alison Langton, who has shown extraordinary patience. Finally, the project would have been impossible without the forbearance and support of our wives and families.

Contents

Part III: General problems

Collaborators

MICHAEL DE SWIET M.D., M.R.C.P. (Chapter 44)
Senior Lecturer,
Cardiothoracic Institute, University of London

ABDULMONEIM EL SEED M.B., M.R.C.P., D.C.H. (Chapter 42)
Associate Professor of Paediatrics
University of Khartoum, Sudan

KIM FOX M.B., M.R.C.P. (Chapter 45)
Research Fellow,
Hammersmith Hospital, London

OWEN D. H. JONES M.B., M.R.C.P. (Appendix)
Registrar,
Brompton Hospital, London

DENNIS KRIKLER M.D., F.R.C.P. (Chapter 45)
Consultant Cardiologist,
Hammersmith Hospital, London

CHRISTOPHER LINCOLN, F.R.C.S. (Chapter 11 and surgical treatment)
Consultant Cardiothoracic Surgeon,
Brompton Hospital, London

MICHAEL L. RIGBY M.B., M.R.C.P. (Appendix)
Senior Registrar,
Brompton Hospital, London

TOM R. TRAILL, M.B., M.R.C.P. (Chapter 9)
Senior Registrar,
Brompton Hospital, London

JAMES R. ZUBERBUHLER, M.D. (Chapters 5, 6, and 12)
Professor of Paediatric Cardiology,
University of Pittsburgh,
Pittsburgh, Pennsylvania, U.S.A.

Part I
Basic considerations

1 Incidence and mortality

The incidence of congenital heart disease in all populations where data are adequate is between 8 and 10 per 1000 live births. The highest mortality from these anomalies occurs during the neonatal period. Until the last 20 years, 25–30 per cent of all children born with congenital heart disease died within the first four weeks of life. In developed countries, up to 15 per cent of all neonatal deaths are attributable to congenital heart disease. With greater understanding of the natural history, anatomy, and physiology, however, recent advances in treatment have radically improved the life expectancy of affected patients, particularly in the neonatal period. Thus, many children with complex anomalies such as transposition of the great arteries will now survive to adult life and will come under the care of general physicians or adult cardiologists. For this reason alone, an account of congenital cardiac anomalies is relevant to all concerned in the treatment and diagnosis of patients with heart disease.

References

Keith, J. D. (1978). In *Heart disease in infancy and childhood* (eds. J. D. Keith, R. D. Rowe, and P. Vlad), p. 3, Macmillan, New York.

Mitchell, S. C., Korones, S. B., and Berendes, H. W. (1971). Congenital heart disease in 56,109 births. *Circulation* **43**, 323.

2 Aetiology

The aetiology of the majority of congenital cardiac anomalies remains unknown. Most cases are sporadic and occur as isolated events in otherwise normal families.

Specific chromosomal abnormalities are associated with cardiac anomalies but account for only a small proportion of all children with congenital heart disease. Thus children with Down's syndrome (mongolism) due to trisomy 21, have a particular propensity for complete or partial (ostium primum) atrioventricular canal defects as well as persistent ductus arteriosus and isolated ventricular septal defect. Similarly, coarctation of the aorta is common in Turner's syndrome (XO complement of chromosomes), whereas the XO/XX mosaic is associated with pulmonary stenosis.

It is recognized that in some families two or more children have similar cardiac malformations and that some pairs of monozygotic or dizygotic twins have the same anomaly. None the less this is not the rule and in several studies of monozygotic twins when one twin was affected, the other was normal. Thus genetic factors alone are rarely causal, although there are families where atrial septal defects, certain cardiomyopathies, or endocardial fibroelastosis are inherited as autosomal dominants (with variable penetrance) or as autosomal recessives.

Specific environmental factors are known to cause cardiac malformations. The best established and most important is infection with rubella virus occurring during the first trimester of the mother's pregnancy. Deafness is the greatest risk to the fetus, then cardiac anomalies. The commonest specific anomaly is persistent ductus arteriosus, followed by ventricular septal defect, Fallot's tetralogy, and peripheral pulmonary stenosis. Maternal rubella is responsible for about 1 per cent of congenital cardiac anomalies. Other viral infections during pregnancy have been incriminated but do not appear to account for many cases of congenital heart disease. Of drugs, thalidomide (peripheral pulmonary stenosis) and some of the cytotoxic agents have been shown to produce cardiac anomalies. Recently, congenital heart block has been shown to be associated with maternal collagen disease such as systemic lupus erythematosus.

References

Nora, J. J. (1968). Multifactorial inheritance hypothesis for the etiology of congenital heart diseases. *Circulation* **38**, 604.

Nora, J. J., Toress, F. G., Sinha, A. K., and McNamara, D. G. (1970). Characteristic cardiovascular anomalies of XO Turner syndrome, XX and XY phenotype and XO/XX Turner mosaic. *American Journal of Cardiology* **25**, 639.

Nora, J. J. (1978). Etiologic aspects of congenital heart disease. In *Heart disease in infants, children and adolescents* (ed. A. J. Moss, F. H. Adams, and G. C. Emmanouilides), pp. 3–11. Williams & Wilkins, Baltimore.

Rowe, R. D., Uchida, I. A., and Char, F. (1978). Heart disease associated with chromosomal abnormalities. In *Heart disease in infancy and childhood* (eds. J. D. Keith *et al.*) pp. 897–925. Macmillan, New York.

Uchida, I. A. (1978). Familial occurrence of congenital heart disease. In *Heart disease in infancy and childhood* (ed. J. D. Keith, *et al.*), pp. 153–9. Macmillan, New York.

3 Nomenclature

For a nomenclature to be of value in modern paediatric cardiology, it must be capable of describing any combination of cardiac malformations which may be encountered. Furthermore, it should, as far as possible, allow for the precise classification of such malformations to be made during the patient's life. At the present time, it is common for given cardiac malformations to be defined as discrete entities. However, complex cardiac malformations are being reported with increasing frequency which do not lend themselves to categorization within these rigid classifications. The majority of paediatric cardiologists are now adopting a concept of nomenclature based upon sequential chamber localization.

In most hearts studied, the sequential chamber arrangement will prove to be normal. That is to say that the right-sided right atrium will connect to the right ventricle which gives rise to the pulmonary artery, and the left atrium will connect to the left ventricle giving rise to the aorta. Such a normal arrangement, however, cannot be assumed until proven. Furthermore, the use of sequential analysis does not complicate description of simple cases yet permits easy and simple categorization of complex malformations.

The system depends upon establishing the morphology and connexions of the cardiac chambers and great arteries, as well as determining the spatial relationships of these structures to each other. The whole approach starts with accurate localization of atrial situs (Figs. 3.1, 3.2).

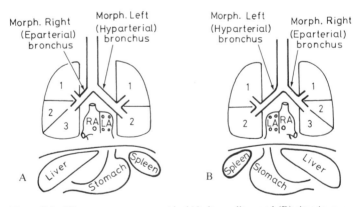

Figure 3.1 The organ arrangement in (A) situs solitus and (B) situs inversus.

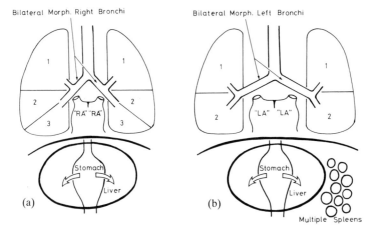

Fig. 3.2 The organ arrangement in situs ambiguus of (a) bilateral right lung type (usually with asplenia) and (b) bilateral left lung type (usually with polysplenia).

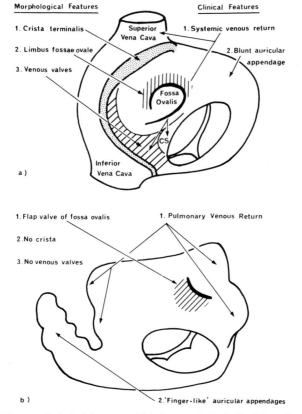

Fig. 3.3 The morphological features of (a) the morphologically right atrium and (b) the morphologically left atrium.

Table 3.1 Possible connexions of the cardiac segments

Atrial situs	Situs solitus
	Situs inversus
	Situs ambiguus
Atrioventricular connexions	Concordant connexion
	Discordant connexion
	Ambiguous connexion
	Double inlet ventricle
	Absence of one AV connexion
Ventriculo-arterial connexions	Concordant connexion
	Discordant connexion
	Double outlet connexion
	Single outlet of the heart

Table 3.2 Ventricular morphology and atrioventricular connexions

Morphology	*Connexion*
Two ventricles	⎰ Concordant
	⎱ Discordant
	Ambiguous
Univentricular heart	
Left ventricular type	⎰ Double inlet
Right ventricular type	⎱ Absence of one AV connexion
Indeterminate type	

Table 3.3 Examples of anomalies which may occur in the various portions of the heart*

Region	Examples of anomalies
Venous return	⎰ Anomalous systemic return
	⎱ Anomalous pulmonary return
Atrial chambers	⎰ Atrial septal defect
	⎱ Cor triatriatum
Atrioventricular junction	⎰ Atrioventricular canal
	⎱ Imperforate AV valve
Ventricular chambers	⎰ Ventricular septal defect
	⎱ Anomalous muscle bundle
Infundibulum and great arteries	⎰ Infundibular septal defect
	⎨ Coarctation
	⎱ Persistent ductus arteriosus

* This is not meant to be an exhaustive catalogue. The anomalies listed are given as examples.

Thereafter, connexions (Table 3.1), spatial relationships, and morphology (Table 3.2) are determined at the atrioventricular and ventriculo-arterial junctions. Once the sequential arrangement has been ascertained, associated anomalies are catalogued throughout the heart, describing anomalies of venous return, malformations of the atria, abnormalities of the atrioventricular junction, malformations of the ventricles, and anomalies of the great arteries (Table 3.3).

Chamber localization

In order to connect the chambers together, it is first necessary to consider how the different cardiac chambers can be recognized in living patients.

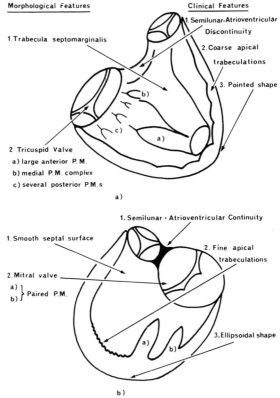

Fig. 3.4 The morphological features of (a) the morphologically right ventricle and (b) the morphologically left ventricle. P.M.: papillary muscle.

Figs. 3.3 and **3.4** are reproduced with permission from Anderson and Shinebourne: *Paediatric Cardiology, 1977*, Churchill Livingstone, Edinburgh.

1. *Morphologically right atrium* (Fig. 3.3a). In the normal heart this chamber receives the systemic venous return. The superior vena cava, inferior vena cava, and coronary sinus enter the smooth-walled sinus venarum, which is separated from the trabeculated right auricle by the prominent crista terminalis. The atrial appendage is typically blunt ending.

2. *Morphologically left atrium* (Fig. 3.3b). This chamber in the normal heart receives the pulmonary venous return through four pulmonary veins. These veins enter a smooth-walled segment which is not separated from the trabeculated auricle by a crista. A characteristic feature of the left atrium is its 'finger-shaped' atrial appendage.

3. *Morphologically right ventricle* (Figs. 3.4a, 3.5A, and 3.6A). In the normal heart this ventricle always possesses an infundibulum and contains the tricuspid valve. Although the leaflet pattern of the tricuspid valve is variable, its papillary muscle pattern of a single anterior muscle, multiple posterior muscles, and a medial papillary muscle is typical. The tricuspid valve is separated from the pulmonary valve by the crista supraventricularis, and a prominent sheet of muscle, the trabecula septomarginalis, is present on the septal surface of the right ventricle. The trabeculations of the right ventricle are coarse.

4. *Morphologically left ventricle* (Figs. 3.4b, 3.5B, and 3.6B). This ventricle contains the easily recognizable bileaflet mitral valve with its paired papillary muscles The mitral valve is in fibrous continuity with the aortic valve; consequently there is no infundibulum. Fine trabeculations are present in the left ventricle.

Plan for sequential analysis
The order of procedure is first to establish atrial situs (Table 3.1). The atrioventricular connexions are then determined (Fig. 3.7) as well as the mode of connexion at the atrioventricular junction (i.e. number and nature of atrioventricular valves—Fig. 3.8). At the same time the morphology of the ventricles or other chambers in the ventricular mass is established (Table 3.2). The ventriculo-arterial connexions are next determined and the morphology of the ventriculo-arterial junction stated (i.e. subaortic, subpulmonary, bilateral, or absent infundibula). Spatial relationships of the cardiac chambers are ascertained and, finally, associated anomalies are catalogued.

1. *Establish atrial situs.* Atrial situs is defined as either *solitus*, *inversus*, or *ambiguus* (Figs. 3.1, 3.2). In situs solitus the morphologically

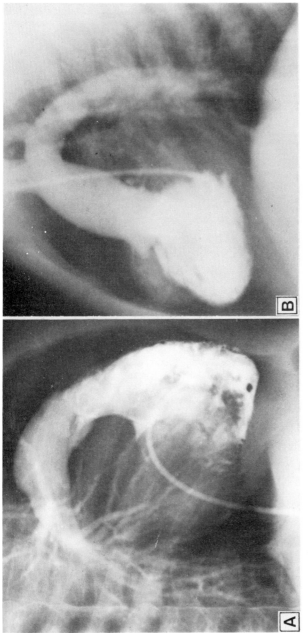

Fig. 3.5 Angiograms illustrating the morphological features of (A) the morphologically right ventricle and (B) the morphologically left ventricle as viewed in the lateral projection.

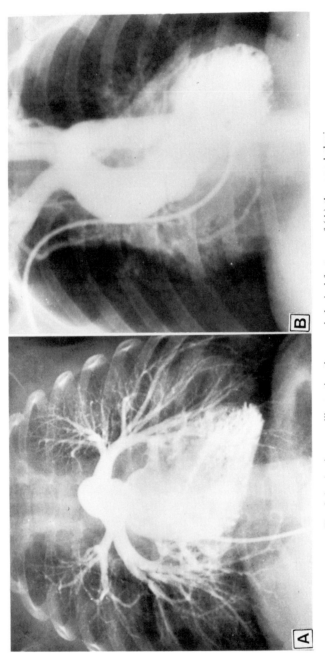

Fig. 3.6 Angiograms illustrating the morphological features of (A) the morphologically right ventricle and (B) the morphologically left ventricle as viewed in the antero-posterior projection.

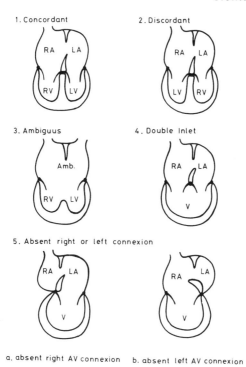

1. Concordant 2. Discordant

3. Ambiguus 4. Double Inlet

5. Absent right or left connexion

a. absent right AV connexion b. absent left AV connexion

Fig. 3.7 The possible types of atrioventricular connexions. Reproduced with permission from Anderson and Shinebourne: *Paediatric Cardiology, 1977*, Churchill Livingstone, Edinburgh.

right atrium is right-sided and the left atrium is left-sided. In situs inversus, the right atrium is left-sided and the left atrium right-sided. In situs ambiguus it is not possible to identify separate right *and* left atria on morphological criteria. Instead, bilaterally symmetrical right (dextro-isomerism) or left (laevo-isomerism) atria and atrial appendages are found. The simplest method of establishing these atrial positions prior to cardiac catheterization is by examination of the plain and penetrated chest radiograph. Thus if the liver is right-sided, inference can usually be made that the inferior vena cava and right atrium are also right-sided, as are the sinus node and tri-lobed morphologically right lung, and that there is *situs solitus* (*solitus* = usual). Conversely, if the liver is left-sided, then the morphologically right atrium (and tri-lobed lung etc.) will usually be left-sided and viscero-atrial *situs inversus* will be present. When the liver is central, then *situs*

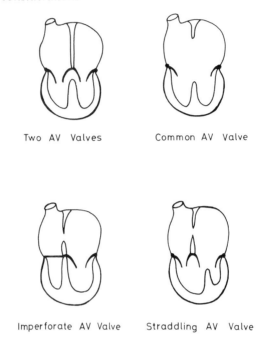

Two AV Valves   Common AV Valve

Imperforate AV Valve   Straddling AV Valve

Fig. 3.8   The different modes of atrioventricular connexion.

ambiguus usually exists, but in difficult cases bronchial anatomy is a better guide to situs ambiguus (Figs. 3.1, 3.2).

2. *Ascertain atrioventricular connexions* (Fig. 3.7). When the morphologically right atrium connects with the morphologically right ventricle and the morphologically left atrium connects with the morphologically left ventricle, then *atrioventricular concordance* is present, irrespective of the ventricular positions within the chest. In contrast, when the morphologically right atrium connects to the morphologically left ventricle and the left atrium to the right ventricle, *atrioventricular discordance* exists, again irrespective of chamber position within the chest. These connexions are established using angiocardiography. The terms concordant and discordant presume the presence of two different identifiable atria and two identifiable ventricles. In the living patient, angiocardiographic criteria for the identification of the morphologically right ventricle (Fig. 3.4a) are the presence of an infundibulum with consequent discontinuity of atrioventricular and arterial valves (Fig. 3.5A) and the triangular shape of the ventricle on the antero-posterior projection (Fig. 3.6A). Criteria for the identification of the morphologically left ventricle (Fig. 3.4b) are absence of an infundibulum, the atrioventricular valve being in fibrous continuity with the arterial valve (Fig. 3.5B), and its ellipsoid shape on both frontal and lateral projections (Figs. 3.5B and 3.6B). In some malformed hearts the morphologically left ventricle may rarely possess an infundibulum. The trabecular pattern of the ventricles is difficult to assess from isolated frames of an angiogram, but on balance the right ventricle, and in particular the septal surface, is more coarsely trabeculated than the left.

In situations where both atrioventricular valves open to the same ventricular chamber, where one atrioventricular valve straddles a septum so that more than half connects to the same ventricle as the other atrioventricular valve, or in the presence of situs ambiguus, the terms concordance and discordance cannot be used. When the two atrioventricular valves (or one plus more than half of a straddling valve) enter the same chamber, the atrioventricular connexion is that of double inlet. If a *double inlet ventricle* is present, then in the terminology used here, there has to be a univentricular heart (see Chapter 22). It is then necessary to describe the ventricular morphology of this univentricular heart (Chapter 22), which may be of left ventricular, right ventricular, or indeterminate type. The presence or absence of a rudimentary chamber (defined as a chamber within the ventricular mass receiving less then half an atrioventricular valve (Chapter 22)) must be determined, and when present its position must also be indicated. Hearts with 'tricuspid atresia' or 'mitral atresia' can also co-exist with ventricular morphologies similar to those seen in double inlet ventricle. These constitute a specific connexion which is *absence of the right or left atrioventricular connexion.* As with double inlet, ventricular morphology and position of the rudimentary chamber must be given so as fully to describe these hearts.

The final instance in which the terms 'concordant' and 'discordant' are inappropriate is in association with situs ambiguus. Situs ambiguus can co-exist with double inlet or absence of one atrioventricular connexion, but when two normally formed ventricles exist, the term *ambiguous atrioventricular connexion* is used, and as in other situations, spatial relationships of the ventricular chambers have to be described (i.e. right ventricle to right or right ventricle to left).

3. *Decide ventriculo-arterial connexions.* As with atrioventricular connexions, this segmental connexion is established by angiocardiography, carried out in a manner which will profile the anterior interven-

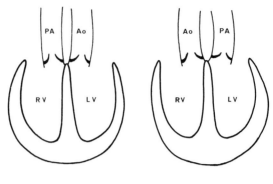

A. CONCORDANT   B. DISCORDANT

Fig. 3.9   The connexions of ventriculo-arterial concordance (A) and ventriculo-arterial discordance (B).
PA   Pulmonary artery
Ao   Aorta
RV   Right ventricle
LV   Left ventricle
Reproduced with permission from Anderson and Shinebourne: *Paediatric Cardiology, 1977,* Churchill Livingstone, Edinburgh.

tricular or trabecular septum. There are four basic patterns in which the great arteries may be connected to their underlying ventricles. These are:

   (a)   arterial concordance (Fig. 3.9A)
   (b)   arterial discordance (Fig. 3.9B)
   (c)   double outlet ventricles (Fig. 3.10)
   (d)   single outlet of the heart (Fig. 3.11).

The first two connexions presuppose identification of two ventricles and a septum (or main chamber and outlet chamber with a trabecular septum) and identification of the ventricular origin of both arteries. In double outlet ventricles more than half of both pulmonary and aortic valves must arise from the same chamber. The term 'single outlet of the heart' describes any situation in which only one great artery can be identified as arising from a ventricle. In defining these connexions, no account is taken of the spatial interrelationships of the arteries which are specified subsequently.

   a. *Arterial concordance* exists when the aorta arises from the morphologically left ventricle (or its rudiment) and the pulmonary artery arises from the morphologically right ventricle (or its rudiment).

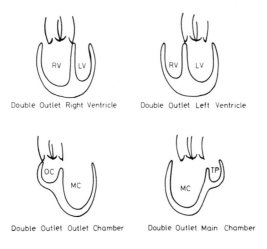

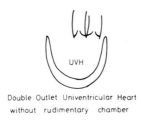

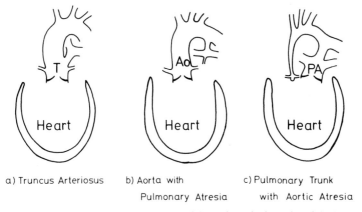

Fig. 3.10 The possible combinations of arteries and chambers giving double outlet ventricles and chambers.

Fig. 3.11 The possible combinations which produce single outlet of the heart.

b. *Arterial discordance* (transposition) is present when the aorta arises from the morphologically right ventricle and the pulmonary artery from the left ventricle (or from the appropriate rudimentary chambers). Thus both great arteries will have been placed across the septum so as to arise from morphologically inappropriate ventricles. Since univentricular hearts without rudimentary chambers do not possess a septum, all arterial connexions in these hearts fall into the double or single outlet categories (see Chapter 22). Since the term 'transposition' describes an abnormal ventriculo-arterial connexion, the terms dextro (*d*) or laevo (*l*) if applied to transposition are used to indicate only the spatial relationship of aortic to pulmonary valve and convey no information regarding atrioventricular connexions. In *d*-transposition the aortic valve is to the right and in *l*-transposition to the left of the pulmonary valve.

c. *Double outlet connexion* (Fig. 3.10). A double outlet connexion is defined as that in which more than half of both great arteries arise from the same ventricle (or outlet chamber).

d. *Single outlet of the heart* (Fig. 3.11). The single trunk can be a truncus arteriosus, an aorta, or a pulmonary trunk, and each may arise from the right ventricle, left ventricle, or in overriding position. The category of single aorta or single pulmonary trunk is used if it is impossible to ascertain the ventricular origin of the other atretic artery. This precludes the necessity of making paradoxical classifications such as 'double outlet right ventricle with pulmonary atresia' or of diagnosing 'transposition with pulmonary atresia' when it is not possible to determine if the pulmonary artery has indeed been placed across the septum. Positive identification of a common arterial trunk (truncus arteriosus) is made when the coronary arteries and one or both pulmonary arteries arise from the ascending portion of a single arterial trunk.

4. *Ascertain relationships.* Right-left and antero-posterior relationships are described usually in terms of the right ventricle being to the right or left of the left ventricle and of the aortic valve being to the right or left of the pulmonary valve. In rare cases the ventricles may bear a supero-inferior relationship.

5. *Tabulate associated anomalies present* (Table 3.3). Any number of anomalies within each segment of the heart can accompany any possible combination of the above connexions. They can be conveniently grouped as:

a anomalies of venous return;
b anomalies of atrial anatomy;
c anomalies of the atrioventricular junction;
d anomalies of ventricular anatomy;
e anomalies of infundibular anatomy; and
f anomalies of the aortic arches and their derivatives.

Cardiac malpositions — dextrocardia, laevocardia, and mesocardia

Having specified connexions and anomalies within the heart, it may be considered desirable to specify the position of the heart within the chest, remembering that this conveys no information about the internal cardiac anatomy or connexions. The heart may be within the right chest, within the left chest, or centrally placed. Similarly, the apex of the heart may point to the left (laevocardia), right (dextrocardia), or not be identifiable (mesocardia). Rotation of the heart about its long axis may also occur. If the present nomenclature is used, positional abnormalities of the heart within the chest will not affect interpretation of the anomaly. In addition, it becomes apparent that terms such as dextrocardia, dextroversion, or dextrorotation add little to the understanding of the anatomy or may even confuse it. (They may, however, help in interpreting an ECG!)

References

Anderson, R. H. and Shinebourne, E. A. (1978). *Paediatric cardiology, 1977*. Chapters 1–4. Churchill Livingstone, Edinburgh.

Brandt, P. W. T. and Calder, A. L. (1977). Cardiac connections: The segmental approach to radiologic diagnosis in congenital heart disease. *Current problems in diagnostic radiology* 7, 1.

Shinebourne, E. A., Macartney, F. J., and Anderson, R. H. (1976). Sequential chamber localisation—logical approach to diagnosis in congenital heart disease. *British Heart Journal* **38**, 327.

Tynan, M. J., Becker, A. E., Macartney, F. J., Quero-Jiminez, M., Shinebourne, E. A., and Anderson, R. H. (1979). The nomenclature and classification of congenital heart disease. *British Heart Journal* **41**, 544.

Van Praagh, R. (1972). Segmental approach to diagnosis in congenital heart disease. In *Birth defects*, pp. 4–23. Williams & Wilkins, Baltimore.

4 Changes in the circulation at birth: Influence of congenital heart disease

There are two ways of approaching the clinical manifestations of congenital heart disease. The first is to consider each congenital anomaly as a discrete entity, and to describe its clinical pattern. Alternatively, attention can be focused upon the principles underlying presentation and symptomatology, and the factors producing each clinical feature can be considered. In this book we will attempt to combine these approaches, dealing first with principles underlying symptomatology, and then describing the clinical features of individual entities in separate chapters.

Congenital cardiac anomalies are not fixed anatomic entities each leading to a predetermined haemodynamic disturbance. The physiology (and anatomy) alter with time, the greatest haemodynamic changes occurring in the first days of life as the infant's circulation adapts from an intra-uterine to an extra-uterine existence. It is therefore essential to understand the normal circulatory changes at birth especially in the younger age groups, and how these are influenced by cardiac malformations.

The fetal circulation

In the fetus, the most highly oxygenated blood (Po_2 roughly equal to 28 mmHg) returns to the right atrium via the umbilical vein, ductus venosus, and inferior vena cava. The majority of this blood passes across the foramen ovale into the left atrium and thence through the left ventricle to the ascending aorta. In contrast, almost all the superior vena caval return (Po_2 roughly equal to 10 mmHg) passes through the right atrium and tricuspid valve to the right ventricle and main pulmonary trunk. Because of the high pulmonary vascular resistance in the fetus (see below), only a small proportion of this blood passes to the lungs, most traversing the ductus arteriosus to reach the descending aorta. As a result of this arrangement, the more highly oxygenated blood is directed to the coronary arteries and the arteries supplying the brain. Blood with the lowest oxygen content passes from the descending aorta to the placenta via the paired umbilical arteries which arise from the internal iliac arteries.

Organ blood flow within the fetus is dependent upon vascular resistance of that organ. Because of the widely patent ductus arteriosus, both ventricles eject blood against effectively the same total vascular resistance. In the normal fetal heart the right ventricle ejects approximately* 60 per cent of the combined ventricular output while the left ventricle ejects 40 per cent. The dimensions of the great arteries are dependent upon flow through them. The total fetal cardiac output is distributed as follows: 40 per cent traverses the ascending aorta, 4 per cent going to the coronary arteries, and 20 per cent to the head and neck arteries. This leaves 16 per cent to traverse the aortic isthmus between the left subclavian artery and the ductus arteriosus. Sixty per cent is ejected through the main pulmonary artery but only 8 per cent passes to the lungs. The remaining 52 per cent passes through the ductus to the descending aorta. The descending aorta, therefore, receives 68 per cent (52 per cent + 16 per cent) of the cardiac output and is considerably larger than the aortic isthmus (16 per cent). Hence, a narrow aortic isthmus is a normal finding in the fetus at term (Fig. 4.1). Following closure of the ductus subsequent to birth, remoulding and expansion of the isthmus occurs, but it is important at this stage not to mistake normal isthmal narrowing for coarctation.

The dimensions of the aorta and pulmonary artery, described above for the normal, may be profoundly influenced by intracardiac anomalies which alter the amounts of blood reaching these arteries. Thus in pulmonary atresia all the fetal cardiac output leaves the heart via the ascending aorta which is large. In this situation, or in any anatomical situation resulting in severe restriction of main pulmonary artery flow in the fetus, aortic isthmal narrowing will not occur. Conversely, if flow to the ascending aorta is limited by intracardiac anomalies such as aortic or subaortic stenosis, the flow will be predominantly directed to a dilated pulmonary artery and the aorta and its isthmus will be small or even severely hypoplastic (see Chapter 38).

Normal circulatory changes at birth

The most important change in the circulation occurs at the moment of birth when the placenta is excluded from the systemic circulation and the lungs expand. Systemic resistance rises abruptly as the pulmonary vascular resistance starts to fall. Pulmonary vascular resistance is high *in utero*, mainly because of constriction of small pulmonary arteries in

* Extrapolated from fetal lamb studies.

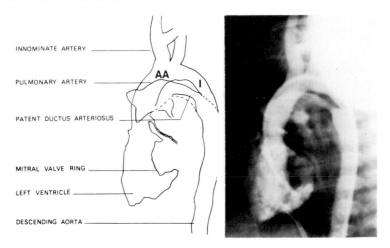

INNOMINATE ARTERY

PULMONARY ARTERY

AA

I

PATENT DUCTUS ARTERIOSUS

MITRAL VALVE RING

LEFT VENTRICLE

DESCENDING AORTA

Fig. 4.1 Left ventricular angiogram viewed in the lateral projection illustrating the dimensions of the ductus arteriosus, isthmus of the aorta (I) and ascending aorta (AA) in a newborn infant.

response to the low arterial oxygen saturation in the fetus. In late pregnancy there is a progressive increase in the medial thickness of these arteries.

At birth the rise in pulmonary arterial oxygen saturation and alveolar Po_2 together with mechanical expansion of the lungs contribute to a reduction in pulmonary vasoconstriction. As the pulmonary vascular resistance falls, so pulmonary blood flow increases. The medial layer of the small pulmonary arteries gradually becomes thinner and by the time the normal full-term infant is 10–14 days old, the pulmonary vascular resistance has fallen to adult level.

Applied physiology of the pulmonary circulation after birth
The rate of fall of pulmonary vascular resistance is delayed principally in two situations. Firstly in the presence of hypoxia and/or hypercapnia. Infants who are hypoxic from lung disease, or who exhibit persistent hypoventilation from cerebral causes for long periods after birth, show a slower rate of fall of pulmonary vascular resistance. Similarly, infants born at high altitude show a delayed fall of resistance compared with those born at sea level and have more muscle in the walls of the small pulmonary arteries.

The second situation is in congenital cardiac anomalies with a large communication between the systemic and pulmonary circulation, such as a persistent ductus arteriosus, ventricular septal defect, or truncus arteriosus. These are all characterized by a potential high-pressure shunt from the systemic to the pulmonary circuit. In these anomalies, however, the amount of blood that is shunted from left-to-right *depends* on the relationship of pulmonary to systemic vascular resistance. They are examples of *dependent* shunts, in contrast to *obligatory* shunts in which the amount of shunting is little affected by the pulmonary vascular resistance (see below). The concepts of dependent and obligatory shunting are illustrated in Fig. 4.2. Infants with large communications and dependent shunts might be expected to go into cardiac failure in the first week of life. However, this is unusual and definite symptoms of congestive heart failure seldom occur before 3–12 weeks. The reason for this relatively late onset is delay in the fall

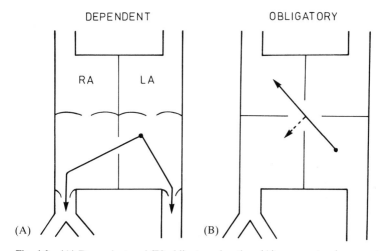

Fig. 4.2 (A) Dependent and (B) obligatory shunting. (A) represents a large ventricular septal defect. During systole both aortic and pulmonary valves are open. The magnitude of the left to right shunt is firstly a function of the size of the defect and secondly of the relative pulmonary and systemic vascular resistances. The lower the ratio of pulmonary to systemic vascular resistance the greater will be the tendency for a red blood cell to pass across the defect and into the pulmonary artery. Thus the magnitude of shunting is *dependent* on the ratio of pulmonary to systemic vascular resistance. (B) represents the situation in an atrioventricular canal defect when there is the possibility for blood to be shunted from left ventricle through a cleft mitral valve across an ostium primum atrial septal defect and into the right atrium. This amounts to a left ventricular to right atrial shunt. As left ventricular pressure is always higher than that in the right atrium the magnitude of shunting is relatively independent of pulmonary vascular resistance i.e. *obligatory*. The dotted line indicates the fact that in atrioventricular canal defects there may be an element of dependent shunting in addition to the dominant obligatory shunt.

of pulmonary vascular resistance together with persistence of the fetal amount of muscle in the media. However, cardiac failure may appear in the first week in premature babies with a dependent shunt. This is in part due to the fact that the muscle in the media of the small pulmonary arteries of these patients is relatively poorly developed at birth and a high pulmonary vascular resistance is not maintained in the face of the systemic pressures transmitted through the defect.

An understanding of the differences between dependent and obligatory shunting helps to rationalize the approach to management of left-to-right shunt situations in congenital heart disease. In obligatory shunts, the anatomy is such that left-to-right shunting occurs irrespective of the relationship between pulmonary and systemic resistance. Such a shunt is that between the left ventricle and the right atrium (Fig. 4.2) in defects of the atrioventricular portion of the membranous ventricular septum (Gerbode defect). As the pressure in the left ventricle is always higher than that in the right atrium, left-to-right shunting will occur irrespective of changes in pulmonary vascular resistance. A similar situation is found in large congenital systemic arteriovenous fistulae and in many atrioventricular canal defects (complete defects or ostium primum atrial septal defect). Whether a shunt is dependent or obligatory is of paramount importance in determining management. For dependent shunts, pulmonary arterial banding to raise the resistance against which the right ventricle ejects blood would be an appropriate (if not necessarily *the* most appropriate) form of management. In contrast, banding an obligatory shunt could prove disastrous since it would increase right ventricular work without diminishing the left-to-right shunt.

Persistent fetal (transitional) circulation

This constitutes a rare syndrome in the newborn in which the heart is structurally normal, the foramen ovale and ductus arteriosus are patent, and the pulmonary vascular resistance remains persistently high. Consequently right-to-left shunting occurs at both atrial and ductal levels with resultant cyanosis. Although no precipitating factors may be identified, infants of diabetic mothers, infants with severe birth asphyxia, and those with a high haematocrit are particularly affected.

Clinical presentation is with cyanosis, often tachypnoea, and sometimes heart failure. The only other abnormality on examination will be a loud pulmonary component to the second sound, although the latter may be difficult to split. The ECG will show the normal neonatal pattern. Chest X-ray will reveal decreased pulmonary vascular marking but may be normal. 100 per cent oxygen does not initially lower the pulmonary vascular resistance and as right-to-left shunting occurs at atrial as well as ductal level, arterial blood gases in 100 per cent oxygen will not exclude cyanotic heart disease (Chapter 6). Differential diagnosis depends on whether it is possible to split the second sound. Thus while some patients are misdiagnosed as complete transposition of the great arteries, in others severe pulmonary outflow tract obstruction will be simulated. Echocardiography helps to clarify the diagnosis but in some cardiac catheterization and angiography are necessary positively to exclude intracardiac anomalies.

Treatment consists of correcting polycythaemia if present and nursing the baby in high concentrations of oxygen to encourage pulmonary vasodilatation. Some centres infuse vasodilator agents such as tolazoline into the pulmonary artery. Many babies recover with conservative management although those who were severely asphyxiated at birth do less well.

References

Dawes, G. S. (1968). *Foetal and neonatal physiology*. Yearbook Medical Publishers, Inc., Chicago.

Rudolph, A. M. (1970). The changes in the circulation after birth: Their importance in congenital heart disease. *Circulation* **41**, 343.

Rudolph, A. M. (1974). *Congenital diseases of the heart*, pp. 1–48. Yearbook Medical Publishers, Inc., Chicago.

Shinebourne, E. A. (1974). Growth and development of the cardiovascular system: Functional development. In *Scientific foundations of paediatrics* (ed. J. A. Davis and J. Dobbing), pp. 198–213. Heinemann, London.

5 History and physical examination

While the advent of cardiac catheterization has revolutionized pre-mortem cardiac diagnosis, it has not made a careful clinical evaluation obsolete. Rather, the clinical examination and invasive study are complementary. Congenital heart disease is usually first suspected because of abnormal findings on physical examination and sometimes a reliable diagnosis can be made from these findings alone. More importantly, clinical findings are the basis for selecting patients for invasive study and are helpful in planning catheterization and angiography. In addition, physical findings are useful in following the natural course of congenital heart disease and in judging the results of surgical repair. In this chapter, the steps in performing an adequate clinical examination will be described together with the physiological basis for certain important physical findings.

History

The history of an infant with congenital heart disease may provide evidence of heart failure or of arterial oxygen unsaturation. Parents should always be asked how their child breathes, how he eats, how well he has gained weight, and whether he has been blue. The infant with early heart failure usually feeds poorly. Typically, he tires after taking a small amount of milk, rests or falls briefly asleep, then is hungry again. As congestive heart failure becomes more severe the infant may stop feeding entirely. If an infant with congenital heart disease is not intensely cyanosed, tachypnoea usually indicates an elevated pulmonary venous pressure most commonly due to large pulmonary blood flow, to left ventricular inflow or outflow obstruction, or to left ventricular myocardial disease. Infants with congenital heart disease may show poor weight gain, but the cardiac anomaly and the slow growth may or may not be causally related. Unless the child is markedly cyanosed or has considerable cardiac enlargement, poor growth is unlikely to be due to the cardiac defect and will not improve after its repair. More specifically, if weight is below the third percentile in a child with congenital heart disease yet head circumference is normal, growth impairment is probably due to the cardiac abnormality. Conversely, if head circumference is also below the third percentile, small stature is unlikely to be due to heart disease.

Parents usually volunteer information about episodes of cyanosis, especially if accompanied by respiratory distress or change in level of consciousness, as in the hypoxaemic (hypercyanotic) spells of tetralogy of Fallot. They may not, however, be aware of even moderate cyanosis if it is constant. In a cyanotic infant it is well to enquire as to the adequacy of intake of iron-containing foods, since relative anaemia can increase symptoms by reducing the oxygen-carrying capacity of the blood. Thus, a child with tetralogy of Fallot may function well at a haemoglobin level of 17 g/dl, yet become quite limited or begin to have hypoxaemic spells with a haemoglobin of 12 g/dl. Anaemia, especially of the microcytic type characteristic of iron deficiency, may precipitate a cerebrovascular accident in a child with cyanotic congenital heart disease as apparent blood viscosity will be increased.

Symptoms may be difficult to evaluate in the older child with a cardiac defect. The child himself may be unaware of or minimize real limitations, while an overconcerned parent may report easy fatigue and exercise intolerance in children with trivial anomalies. In children, chest pain is very rarely of cardiac origin and the worried parent should be told this. The truly symptomatic child virtually always has other evidence of the severity of his anomaly on physical examination, chest X-ray, or electrocardiogram. If cardiac symptoms seem out of proportion it is often helpful to observe the child during exercise.

Physical examination

Two prerequisites of a good physical examination are a quiet environment and a cooperative child. Neither is always easy to obtain. In hospital, the television and garrulous colleagues are common offenders. Both should be turned off.

The young infant who is fed and dry is usually quiet. The two-year-old may not be. At this age a child is often most easily examined in his mother's lap or arms, his attention distracted by a toy or by looking out of the window. He will often feel less attacked by a stethoscope if he examines it first or if his leg or arm or abdomen are 'listened to' first. A smiling examiner is often more tolerable to a frightened child than a solemn one.

1. *Arterial pulses.* An evaluation of peripheral arterial pulses is an important part of the cardiac physical examination. Either the brachial, axillary, or radial pulse should be felt in each arm and compared to a leg pulse. Traditionally the femorals are felt, although infants as well as older children may better tolerate gentle palpation of a dorsalis pedis pulse. If leg pulses are decreased or absent, coarctation of the aorta is present. However, since femoral pulses may seem diminished even in the normal chubby infant or obese older child it is well to check dorsalis pedis or posterior tibial pulses before concluding that coarctation indeed exists. The origin of the left subclavian artery may or may not be involved in the coarctation and pulses in the left arm can resemble leg pulses, the right arm pulse, or be intermediate. A delay in the femoral pulse is common with coarctation of the aorta and can be identified by feeling a major arm pulse and femoral pulse simultaneously. In the older child with coarctation, arterial collaterals are often present, particularly over the posterior thorax in the periscapular areas. They may be located by running the hand lightly over the back or by viewing the back obliquely from one side with the light source on the opposite side.

Leg pulses are variable in the presence of an interrupted aortic arch. If the ductus arteriosus, which in this entity is the source of blood supply to the lower body, is widely open, pulmonary pressure will be transmitted to the descending aorta and leg pulses will be easily felt. If the ductus is constricted, only a damped pressure will be transmitted, pulse pressures will be small, and leg pulses weak or absent.

If all peripheral arterial pulses are poor in an infant, left ventricular outflow is likely to be very low, either because of obstruction (severe aortic stenosis or aortic atresia) or depressed myocardial function. Pulses are increased when pulse pressure is widened by a low resistance run-off from the systemic arterial system (persistent ductus arteriosus, aorto-pulmonary window, truncus arteriosus, systemic arterio-venous fistula) or by aortic regurgitation. Pulses may also be increased when myocardial inotropy is high and most of the stroke volume is ejected in early systole (as in hypertrophic cardiomyopathy) and are also increased with fever and with physical exercise. Prominent suprasternal notch pulsations are common with coarctation and with aortic regurgitation, and in the paediatric age group a pulsatile mass just lateral to the suprasternal notch suggests a cervical loop aorta. Striking respiratory variation in pulse amplitude suggest pericardial tamponade and is dealt with further in the discussion on blood pressure.

2. *Blood pressure.* Blood pressure determination is an integral part of the cardiac physical examination. Ideally, pressure should be measured in both arms and a leg, and this is mandatory if coarctation of the aorta is suspected. For accurate blood pressure determination the cuff must be of adequate width, covering at least two-thirds of the upper arm from elbow to axilla, and the rubber tourniquet must completely encircle the arm. (A small or loosely attached cuff leads to spuriously high blood pressure determinations.) As the cuff is inflated and then deflated, Korotkoff sounds appear at systolic blood pressure and abruptly change intensity (or disappear, whichever comes first) at diastolic blood pressure. Use of the Doppler technique to measure systolic blood pressure greatly facilitates the measurement and is the most accurate noninvasive technique. The 'flush' method of determining blood pressure in infants variably underestimates the true reading and is not advised, as blood pressure can be obtained by auscultation or palpation even in the absence of a Doppler probe.

Elevated blood pressure may be due to coarctation of the aorta, renal parenchymal disease, renal artery stenosis, or may have no demonstrable aetiology (essential hypertension, see Chapter 44). Low blood pressure is rarely of significance unless the infant is obviously ill and has a low cardiac output. Asymmetry of blood pressure levels is most often due to coarctation of the aorta, blood pressure in the legs being lower than blood pressure in the right arm. Pressure in the left arm may be high or low depending upon whether the left subclavian artery is involved in the coarctation. Blood pressure is often lower in the left arm than in the right in supravalvar aortic stenosis.

Arterial blood pressure normally varies slightly with respiration, falling with inspiration and rising with expiration. If this respiratory variation is exaggerated it is described as 'paradoxical'. Exaggerated variations may occur with airway obstruction, with its attendant wide swings in intrathoracic pressure, with congestive heart failure, or with pericardial tamponade. To identify and quantify a 'paradoxical' pulse, the blood pressure cuff is inflated until Korotkoff sounds are not heard in any phase of the respiratory cycle, then slowly deflated until sounds appear during expiration. The cuff is further deflated until sounds appear during inspiration as well. The difference, in mmHg, between the appearance of Korotkoff sounds in expiration and their presence throughout the respiratory cycle is a measure of the 'paradoxical' pulse or blood pressure. A difference greater than 10 mmHg is abnormal and if the difference is greater than 20 mmHg, tamponade is likely.

3. *The jugular venous pulse.* The jugular venous pulse is less emphasized by paediatric cardiologists than by cardiologists dealing with an adult population. Neck veins are hard to see in infants, and liver enlargement and tachypnoea are usually better indicators of congestive heart failure. In the setting of congestive heart failure during infancy, grossly distended neck veins suggest the possibility of an intra-cranial arterio-venous fistula.

Visible pulsations in the jugular veins may be venous waves or transmitted impulses from the carotid arteries. Transmitted arterial pulsations can be identified if venous waves are damped by light pressure over the jugular veins just above the clavicle. In infants this is best accomplished by stretching the skin over this area. Venous pulsations may be A-waves, signifying impedance to exit of blood from the right atrium. They are exaggerated in tricuspid atresia when the interatrial communication is small and restrictive, and with very severe right ventricular outflow tract obstruction if the ventricular septum is intact. With complete atrioventricular block large 'cannon' waves are generated when atrial and ventricular systole coincide, the atrium then contracting against a closed tricuspid valve. Large A-waves may also occur with hypertrophic cardiomyopathy. Large V-waves may be seen with severe tricuspid regurgitation. Large A and V-waves may be palpable over the jugular veins and also below the right costal margin (as hepatic pulsations).

4. *Precordial motion.* Abnormal precordial motion may be either seen or felt. Right ventricular overactivity causes a rather sustained systolic outward movement along the left sternal border (parasternal heave). It is most marked when there is both pressure and volume overload of this chamber. Volume overload of the left ventricle, as with severe mitral regurgitation, causes a less sustained early systolic outward movement at the apex. An aneurysm of the right ventricular outflow tract, usually the result of excessive resection of infundibular muscle or of patching the outflow tract during tetralogy of Fallot repair, can cause a visible and palpable systolic bulge at the mid and high left sternal border. A palpable presystolic outward movement at the apex may accompany a loud fourth heart sound, most commonly with hypertrophic cardiomyopathy.

5. *Heart sounds.* One cannot simply clap a stethoscope to a patient's chest and hope for the best, waiting expectantly for diagnosis to flow unbidden through the stethoscope tubing to the brain. Patience, a systematic approach, and knowledge of the pathophysiology of congenital cardiac lesions each increase the yield of auscultation. There are certain classic auscultatory areas where sounds and murmurs of importance are most likely to be heard. These are the high right sternal border, the high, mid and low left sternal border, and the apex. Each must be examined in turn. The cardiac cycle is made of systole and diastole, separated by the first and second heart sounds. It cannot be listened to as a whole but must be dissected into these parts, each then being individually examined.

The precise origin of the first and second heart sounds is still debated. Do they arise from the cardiac valves themselves or from the sudden checking of a column of blood in proximity to the valves? In either event the sounds coincide temporally with valve closure. The first heart sound is generated as tricuspid and mitral valves close. Normally, mitral valve closure follows so closely after tricuspid that the first heart sound is single to the ear, although tricuspid and mitral components may be identified by phonocardiography. The mitral closure sound is usually louder than the tricuspid, the first heart sound thus being loudest at the apex. If the tricuspid closure sound is accentuated, the first heart sound may be louder at the low left sternal border.

The loudness of the first heart sound is influenced by the position of the valve leaflets as ventricular systole begins and by the velocity of their closure. If they are wide open, closure will be during the rapid phase of ventricular pressure rise and will be forceful and loud. Thus, for instance, if the P–R interval is short, the flow occasioned by atrial contraction will keep the atrioventricular valves open until ventricular systole begins. The first heart sound will then be loud. The increased late diastolic mitral blood flow of mitral stenosis also results in a loud first heart sound, the mitral component being accentuated. The loud first sound commonly associated with an interatrial septal defect is loudest at the low left sternal border, suggesting that a loud tricuspid component may be responsible. Here, total tricuspid diastolic flow is increased and rapid flow may extend into late diastole resulting in tricuspid valve closure during the rapid phase of right ventricular pressure rise.

In contrast, valves that have floated towards the closed position at the onset of systole, for example after a prolonged P–R interval, will produce a soft first heart sound. A soft first heart sound may also be present if myocardial contractility is greatly impaired, as with severe myocarditis or cardiomyopathy.

The second heart sound is coincident with aortic and pulmonary valve closure. During auscultation it is of paramount importance to determine if two components are present. If they are clearly heard, the presence of both arterial valves is established. If the second sound is single, one arterial valve may be atretic or its closure may be so soft as to be inaudible. If two components are present but are separated by 20 ms or less, the second sound will seem single to the ear. Although the aortic closure sound is widely transmitted the pulmonary sound is localized and a 'split' second sound is usually most easily heard at the high or mid left sternal border, occasionally being audible at the high right sternal border. A 'split second sound' heard only at the low left sternal border or apex is more likely to be caused by a third heart sound (protodiastolic gallop) or by an opening snap (mitral) following an aortic closure sound.

If two components of the second sound are present, it is most important to examine the effect of respiration on the temporal relationship of these two sounds. During inspiration pulmonary closure normally occurs after aortic closure, as systemic venous return and hence right ventricular stroke volume increase and termination of right ventricular ejection is delayed. Thus, during inspiration the second sound has two audible components and is 'split'. With expiration systemic venous return decreases, causing right ventricular stroke volume and ejection period to decrease and the pulmonary closure sound to occur earlier. There is also an increase in pulmonary venous return, causing aortic valve closure to be slightly delayed. Aortic and pulmonary closure thus coincide and the second sound becomes single during expiration.

Splitting may be abnormally wide (over 60 ms) if right ventricular stroke volume is very large, if there is a delay in right ventricular mechanical events due to right bundle branch block, or if the right ventricular ejection period is prolonged by outflow tract obstruction. If there is no variation in the separation of aortic and pulmonary closure sounds during respiration, the second sound is said to be 'fixedly' split. Fixed splitting is characteristic of an atrial septal defect, the large communication between the atria ensuring near equality of right and left atrial pressures. Thus, although systemic and pulmonary venous return continue to vary with respiration, relative right and left ventricular filling remains constant as does the temporal relationship between aortic and pulmonary closure.

Paradoxical splitting occurs when the pulmonary closure sound precedes the aortic sound, the split widening with expiration and disappearing with inspiration. The usual cause is a delay in aortic closure occasioned by left bundle branch block, severe left ventricular outflow obstruction or left ventricular dysfunction. Paradoxical splitting can also result from the premature right ventricular events associated with Type B Wolff–Parkinson–White syndrome.

Fixed or paradoxical splitting may be evident during quiet respiration but can perhaps be better defined during held expiration. The child is asked to breathe in, to breathe out, and then to stop breathing. Normally, the second sound is single for two or more beats following end expiration, then splits narrowly and subsequently more widely as systemic venous return gradually increases. With fixed splitting, the second sound is split even at end expiration and the width of split is constant as the breath is held. If splitting is paradoxical, the second sound is split at end expiration and becomes single over the next few beats.

The loudness of the pulmonary valve closure sound is a vitally important piece of information but cannot be gauged until the pulmonary component of the second sound is identified with certainty. For example, a loud single second heart sound at the high left sternal border is not necessarily a loud pulmonary closure sound. It may instead represent closure of an abnormally positioned aortic valve (as in, for example, complete transposition or tetralogy of Fallot). Once respiratory variation has been determined, aortic and pulmonary closure sounds can be distinguished. With normal, wide, or fixed splitting, the pulmonary closure sound is always the second component of the sound. With paradoxical splitting, the pulmonary sound is the first component. The loudness of the pulmonary closure sound has several determinants including the position of the valve within the thorax, structures interposed between the valve and the stethoscope, and the pulmonary artery pressure at the start of diastole. Thus the pulmonary closure sound at the high left sternal border is loud with pulmonary hypertension, but also may be loud in the thin-chested child. While the low pulmonary artery diastolic pressure occasioned by right ventricular outflow tract obstruction tends to make pulmonary closure soft or inaudible, so does a posterior location of the pulmonary valve, as in complete transposition.

A third heart sound is coincident with rapid early diastolic ventricular filling and is commonly heard in normal children. The usual gallop heard in children with congestive heart failure is either an accentuated third sound or a summation of third and fourth sounds as tachycardia shortens diastole.

Early systolic ejection sounds may have a pulmonary or aortic origin. A pulmonary ejection sound may emanate from a stenotic pulmonary valve or from a dilated pulmonary artery. The sound is maximal at the high left sternal border, is high-pitched and is usually distinctly louder during expiration. An aortic ejection sound originates at an abnormal aortic valve or in a dilated aorta. It is often loudest at the apex rather than in the second right intercostal space and unlike a pulmonary ejection sound does not vary with respiration. It is of medium pitch. A mid-systolic click is most commonly associated with a prolapsing mitral valve and is often followed by a late apical systolic murmur. Both click and murmur may be intermittent.

6. *Heart murmurs*. Murmurs should be described in terms of timing, location, loudness, pitch, and quality. Although systole and diastole may seem obvious on auscultation, the timing of a murmur can best be assured by simultaneously feeling a central pulse. Pansystolic (holosystolic) murmurs extend from the first to the second heart sound and are usually plateau-shaped. Ejection systolic murmurs are crescendo-decrescendo and usually end before the second sound. Diastolic murmurs may be early, mid, or late in diastole. The murmurs of aortic regurgitation and of 'hypertensive' pulmonary regurgitation are early diastolic. The murmur of 'normotensive' pulmonary regurgitation begins sometimes after aortic closure and may appear mid-diastolic if pulmonary closure is silent. The murmurs associated with large diastolic flow across the mitral or tricuspid valves are mid-diastolic, with a distinct gap between the second sound and the beginning of the murmur, and are heard with large left-to-right shunts or with severe mitral or tricuspid regurgitation. The typical murmur of mitral stenosis has a late diastolic accentuation due to left atrial systole and hence disappears if atrial fibrillation ensues. A murmur is termed 'continuous' if it extends through the second sound, but it need not occupy all of the cardiac cycle.

A thrill may accompany a loud murmur. Like murmurs, thrills should be carefully timed since they can be diastolic, systolic, or continuous. The presence of a thrill depends not only on the loudness of the murmur but also on its pitch, high-pitched murmurs being less likely to have a thrill.

References

Leatham, A. (1970). *Auscultation of the heart and phonocardiography*. Churchill Livingstone, London.

Leon, D. F. and Shaver, J. A. (1975). *Physiologic principles of heart sounds and murmurs*. AHA Monograph No. 46, The American Heart Association, Inc., New York.

6 Modes of presentation and differential diagnosis of the infant with congenital heart disease

As far as the infant with congenital heart disease is concerned, it must be stressed that specific anatomical diagnosis can frequently not be made *with certainty* on the basis of physical examination, ECG, and chest X-ray alone. Cyanosis, heart failure, or a combination of both are the principal modes of presentation. In certain conditions such as hypoplasia of the left heart (see Chapter 26) shock due to a severely decreased cardiac output is the presenting feature. Alternatively, and commonly, heart disease may be detected because of a heart murmur in an otherwise asymptomatic infant. Less commonly, cardiomegaly may be detected on chest X-ray. In older children it is often easier to make a specific clinical diagnosis, and in this group modes of presentation will be dealt with principally under specific entities.

Cyanosis in congenital heart disease

Cyanosis is a blue discoloration of the mucous membranes due to presence of more than 5 g/dl circulating reduced haemoglobin. Clinical detection of cyanosis depends, therefore, in part on the total haemoglobin concentration. Thus 40 per cent desaturation (or a 60 per cent arterial oxygen saturation) will cause cyanosis in a child with haemoglobin concentration of more than 13 g/dl. If, however, the haemoglobin concentration were below 10 g/dl cyanosis would not be clinically detectable as there would be only 4 g/dl of circulating reduced haemoglobin.

Clinical assessment of cyanosis (or more specifically of arterial desaturation) is therefore inaccurate. Many forms of cyanotic heart disease with right-to-left shunt, but increased pulmonary blood flow (e.g. univentricular hearts or truncus arteriosus) may achieve oxygen saturations at which cyanosis is undetectable. Furthermore, infants with 'acyanotic' cardiac anomalies may become cyanosed when heart failure or a chest infection is present. Similarly, primary lung disease may mimic cyanotic congenital heart disease, especially in the neonatal period; children with polycythaemia may appear cyanosed, and reduced respiratory drive due to central nervous system depression may also cause cyanosis.

To resolve the question as to whether or not a patient has cyanotic congenital heart disease, 100 per cent oxygen should be administered to the infant for 5–10 minutes. If (right)* radial arterial blood samples are taken whilst oxygen administration continues, a Po_2 value of more than 250 mmHg effectively excludes cyanotic heart disease and values of more than 160 mmHg make it unlikely. Failure of Po_2 to rise to this level would be strongly suggestive of cyanotic heart disease, even if levels of 150 mmHg were encountered, a situation in which the child's mucous membranes would appear pink.

Causes of cyanotic congenital heart disease and approach to clinical diagnosis
Cyanosis occurs
  a with right-to-left shunting of blood and reduced pulmonary flow;
  b in the presence of complete transposition of the great arteries;
  c in common mixing situations.

The chest X-ray is the primary ancillary aid in differential diagnosis. A distinction is made between those conditions with definitely diminished pulmonary vascular markings (pulmonary oligaemia) and those with normal or increased pulmonary vascular markings (pulmonary plethora).

Conditions with pulmonary oligaemia on chest X-ray
These patients will be blue because part or all of the systemic venous return is frustrated in its attempt to reach the lungs and is shunted from the right side of the heart to the left. For this to occur, in addition to obstruction to pulmonary blood flow there must be a defect through which the right-to-left shunt occurs. The obstruction may be at tricuspid valve, infundibular or pulmonary valve level, or, more rarely, within the body of the right ventricle or at peripheral pulmonary artery level. Finally, a very high pulmonary vascular resistance where the

---

*Especially in the newborn the ductus arteriosus may be patent. If the pulmonary vascular resistance is elevated, for instance due to lung disease, there will be a right-to-left shunt through the ductus resulting in lower body arterial desaturation. A low Po_2 in femoral arterial blood may thus reflect lung disease rather than cyanotic heart disease. For this reason a radial artery sample is used and the right radial preferred as its origin is normally furthest removed from the ductus. The other circumstances where arterial saturation in 100 per cent oxygen may not reflect cyanotic congenital heart disease are in severe lung disease, when usually the Po_2 will also be elevated, or with persistent transitional fetal circulation (see Chapter 46).

obstruction is in the small pulmonary arteries may cause a reduction in pulmonary flow. The defect may be in the atrial septum, the ventricular septum, or between the great arteries. In the newborn, any obstructive right-sided lesion may produce cyanosis as the foramen ovale provides a route for a right-to-left shunt.

Clinical differential diagnosis: If right ventricular outflow tract obstruction is complete (pulmonary atresia) pulmonary blood flow will be via a patent ductus arteriosus or by systemic–pulmonary collateral arteries. In both a continuous murmur may be audible, usually localized to the second left intercostal space with patent ductus arteriosus, but being more widely distributed and more easily heard with collateral arteries. With mild or moderate pulmonary stenosis an ejection systolic murmur maximal at the second left intercostal space is heard but this disappears with increasing pulmonary outflow tract obstruction, especially when there is no interventricular septum (univentricular heart) or a large ventricular septal defect (tetralogy of Fallot). In the latter situation more of the stroke volume traverses the ventricular septal defect and less passes to the pulmonary artery, the systolic murmur being absent during hypercyanotic spells.

With severe or complete pulmonary outflow tract obstruction pulmonary closure is not audible and the second sound is single. If the second sound is split and the pulmonary component not accentuated in an infant with cyanosis and decreased pulmonary vascular markings, Ebstein's anomaly or Uhl's anomaly, congenital tricuspid incompetence, or a hypoplastic right ventricle should be considered.

On chest X-ray a right aortic arch, pulmonary artery bay (concave upper left cardiac border), and an enlarged ascending aorta suggest tetralogy of Fallot (Fig. 7.1) or pulmonary atresia with ventricular septal defect. Many of the conditions characterized by decreased pulmonary vascular markings on chest X-ray have right ventricular hypertrophy on ECG, usually with a mean frontal QRS axis above $+90°$ (i.e. tetralogy of Fallot, pulmonary atresia plus ventricular septal defect, complete transposition plus ventricular septal defect). If the ECG shows a superior QRS axis lying between 0 and $-90°$ with left ventricular preponderance the probable diagnosis is a univentricular heart of left ventricular type and pulmonary stenosis or atresia, often with absent right atrioventricular connexion (tricuspid atresia); a superior axis, right atrial hypertrophy, and left ventricular dominance are the classical features of 'tricuspid atresia'.

The other anomaly with pulmonary oligaemia on chest X-ray and left ventricular dominance on ECG is pulmonary atresia (or critical pulmonary stenosis) and intact interventricular septum, where the right ventricle, though thickened, has a very small cavity. In both these and some univentricular hearts the mean frontal QRS axis may be inferior and right-sided.

Conditions with normal or increased pulmonary vascular markings on chest X-ray
The entities in this group are complete transposition of the great arteries, the commonest cause of cyanotic heart disease in the newborn period, and common mixing situations. By a common mixing situation is meant the situation in which there is obligatory mixing of the pulmonary and systemic venous returns, the admixed blood being distributed to both pulmonary and systemic arteries. The mixing can occur at atrial, ventricular, or great arterial level. Examples of the former are total anomalous pulmonary venous drainage and common atrium. In univentricular hearts or double outlet ventricles mixing occurs at ventricular level. Truncus arteriosus produces mixing at arterial level. Although pulmonary plethora characterizes the majority of common mixing situations, co-existent obstruction to pulmonary blood flow would produce oligaemic lung fields. Thus in double outlet right ventricle with pulmonary stenosis, cyanosis and oligaemia will be present despite the common mixing situation. Those patients with common mixing and increased pulmonary blood flow will tend to present with both cyanosis and heart failure, as will those with complete transposition of the great arteries complicated by a large ventricular septal defect or persistent ductus arteriosus. Aortic atresia (hypoplastic left heart syndrome) is another example of a common mixing situation, the characteristic features of which are dealt with elsewhere (see Chapter 26).

Clinical differential diagnosis: Clinical differentiation between the entities in this group is not always possible although the added use of echocardiography has considerably enhanced pre-catheter diagnosis. If cyanosis is severe ($Po_2 < 30$ mmHg in 100 per cent oxygen) complete transposition is the probable diagnosis, whereas this anomaly alone is unlikely if the Po_2 rises above 50 mmHg. Extreme tachypnoea is a feature of pulmonary venous obstruction, as in obstructed total anomalous pulmonary venous drainage, or the hypoplastic left heart syndrome. Peripheral pulses are increased with persistent truncus arteriosus; otherwise, with the exception of aortic atresia, they are usually normal in this group of anomalies. On auscultation a split second sound excludes truncus arteriosus (or aortic atresia); most anomalies in this group have a split second sound with an accentuated pulmonary component as well as systolic murmurs which are not particularly helpful in differential diagnosis. However, a continuous murmur is occasionally heard in mitral atresia, being generated at a restrictive interatrial communication, and, occasionally with total anomalous pulmonary venous return, originating at a site of pressure drop within the anomalous channel. Truncal incompetence has systolic and early diastolic murmurs that may merge to become continuous.

Cyanosis with increased pulmonary vascular markings on chest X-ray and *no* heart murmurs is most common in complete transposition of the great arteries but is sometimes found with total anomalous pulmonary venous drainage. The 'characteristic' X-ray of complete transposition of the great arteries, with its narrow pedicle and 'egg-shaped' heart is useful if present, but is not seen in the majority of patients with transposition. A right aortic arch suggests persistent truncus arteriosus in this group, but pulmonary atresia with VSD and excessive pulmonary blood flow via systemic–pulmonary collateral arteries must also be considered.

On ECG, complete transposition and total anomalous pulmonary venous drainage have marked right ventricular forces whereas univentricular hearts of left ventricular type will have dominant left or posterior forces (± a superior mean frontal QRS axis). Most other anomalies in this group with cyanosis and pulmonary plethora on chest X-ray tend to have biventricular or less marked right ventricular hypertrophy.

Heart failure in congenital heart disease
Heart failure in infancy presents as tachypnoea, difficulty in feeding, or as failure to thrive and gain weight. The other principal cause of tachypnoea is lung disease. Infants in heart failure are often thought initially to have a chest infection. Less frequent causes of tachypnoea are cerebral abnormalities and acidosis resulting from renal failure or other metabolic disorders.

Signs
Tachypnoea, tachycardia, and hepatomegaly are the commonest signs of heart failure in infancy and childhood. The clinical features are shown in Table 6.1 together with their pathophysiological basis. Heart failure in infancy differs somewhat from failure in adults. Since the

Table 6.1   Clinical features of heart failure in infancy

Features	Pathophysiological basis
Tachypnoea Dyspnoea/subcostal recession Wheeze Basal crepitations	Pulmonary venous congestion
Hepatomegaly Oedema	Systemic venous congestion
Tachycardia Pallor Sweating Cold extremities Poor pulses	Low cardiac output Increased sympathetic activity
Abnormal weight gain Failing urinary output Evidence of pulmonary and systemic venous congestion	Fluid retention

bronchial tree is of smaller calibre, further narrowing of the lumen by venous congestion of the mucosa will rapidly lead to airways obstruction, diminished alveolar ventilation, and trapping of secretions. Thus expiratory or even inspiratory wheezing is common and CO_2 retention may result. Similarly, bronchopneumonia and recurrent chest infections are common in infants with heart failure, as is difficulty in feeding. Peripheral oedema is the exception in babies. Swollen ankles are more likely to suggest lymphoedema (as in Turner's syndrome) than heart failure. Occasionally peri-orbital oedema is seen in babies. Fluid retention in infants and children usually expresses itself as hepatomegaly as well as by an abnormal weight gain.

Causes
In acyanotic congenital heart disease, three main groups of lesion are responsible:
  a obstructive 'left-sided lesions' which impede forward flow of blood into the systemic circuit;
  b large communications between the systemic and pulmonary circulations (left-to-right shunts);
  c myocardial disease.

Other causes of heart failure to be considered in acyanotic infants are mitral or aortic incompetence, paroxysmal supraventricular tachycardia, arterio-venous fistulae, anaemia (haemolytic disease of the newborn), septicaemia, and overtransfusion.

Cyanotic congenital heart disease may also be accompanied by heart failure (see above) and this must always be excluded by arterial blood gas sampling in 100 per cent oxygen (see p. 36).

In acyanotic infants the commonest cause of heart failure in the first week of life is coarctation of the aorta. Myocardial disease and aortic stenosis are less frequent causes in the first week of life. Patients with *dependent* left-to-right shunts (see p. 23), even with large defects and potentially large shunts, tend to present in heart failure after the first two weeks of life and up to the second month. Those with obligatory shunts may present earlier.

Clinical differential diagnosis
In many of these lesions the diagnosis can be established clinically. Thus, coarctation of the aorta is diagnosed from a discrepancy between upper and lower limb pulses or blood pressures. Palpation of femoral pulses is mandatory in the evaluation of all infants or children, especially of neonates in heart failure, and pressures should if possible be measured in upper and lower limbs using an ultrasonic Doppler technique. Generally decreased pulses can be seen in advanced heart failure of any aetiology but are more characteristic of aortic stenosis and, to a lesser degree, of myocardial disease. In the acyanotic infant, increased pulses are most commonly due to a persistent ductus arteriosus. This entity rarely causes heart failure during the first month, except in the premature infant, and very early heart failure with full pulses should suggest a systemic arterio-venous fistula. Auscultation over the head or liver may disclose a continuous bruit and, with an intracranial fistula, neck veins may be quite dilated, a rare finding with other causes of failure in early infancy. A pulsatile fontanelle and rapidly growing head circumference are other clues. Although discussed here as an acyanotic anomaly, an intracranial or arteriovenous fistula may cause cyanosis as part of the huge systemic venous return crosses the foramen ovale with worsening right ventricular failure.

After one month of age the most common cause of heart failure is increased pulmonary blood flow, usually as a result of left-to-right shunting at ventricular (ventricular septal defect) or great artery level (persistent ductus arteriosus, aorto-pulmonary window). The characteristic murmurs are discussed under the specific anomalies. Shunting occurs at both atrial and ventricular levels with a complete atrioventricular canal, and heart failure may be aggravated by the mitral regurgitation which is common in this anomaly.

In infants with heart failure the chest X-ray typically shows cardiomegaly and often increased pulmonary vascular markings. Notable exceptions in the acyanotic group are mitral stenosis and supraventricular tachycardia. In each the chest X-ray may show pulmonary oedema in the absence of cardiomegaly. The pulmonary oedema of supraventricular tachycardia is probably due to impedance to left atrial emptying, induced by the very short diastolic filling period. Poor ventricular filling may be aggravated in the neonate by a high haemoglobin level and a consequent increase in blood viscosity.

The ECG may be useful in leading to a suspicion of certain rare cardiac anomalies which produce heart failure. Glycogen storage disease of the heart (Pompe's) regularly causes severe heart failure and death in infancy. The ECG typically shows a short P–R interval and left ventricular hypertrophy with or without 'strain'. Anomalous origin of the left coronary artery is usually first suspected when an infarction pattern is seen on the electrocardiogram of an infant in failure, but should also be considered in an infant with otherwise unexplained heart failure who has left ventricular hypertrophy on the ECG.

References

Jones, R. S., Baumer, H., Joseph, M. C., and Shinebourne, E. A. (1976). Arterial oxygen tension and the response to oxygen breathing in the differential diagnosis of congenital heart disease in infancy. *Archives of Diseases of Childhood* **51**, 667.

Talner, N. S., Sanyal, S. K., Halloran, K. H., Gardner, T. H., and Ordway, N. K. (1965). Congestive heart failure in infancy: I. Anomalies in blood gases and acid–base equilibrium. *Paediatrics* **35**, 20.

7 Investigations: the chest X-ray

In practical terms the postero-anterior film provides virtually all the information that can be gleaned from plain chest X-ray and little additional information is gained from oblique or even lateral films. To rule out an anomalous origin of the subclavian artery, barium swallows are routinely performed in many American centres, but this is not the case in England.

When considering the postero-anterior film, it is first necessary to confirm that the patient is not rotated relative to the X-ray tube, as minor degrees of rotation will throw normal structures into undue prominence. Penetration and the technical quality of the film are next assessed, as too soft or pale a film can give a spurious impression of increased pulmonary vascular markings (plethora), whereas overexposure may erroneously suggest pulmonary oligaemia.

Specific analysis then proceeds with examination of the skeleton. Previous operations may give asymmetrical appearances. Rib-notching, typically on the undersurface of the fourth and fifth ribs posteriorly can be found with coarctation in older children. Unilateral rib-notching may similarly be caused by collateral arteries following a Blalock–Taussig (subclavian to pulmonary artery) anastomosis.

Viscero-atrial situs is next assessed, the liver almost always being the same side as the right atrium (Fig. 3.1). The bronchial anatomy, which can be assessed from a penetrated film, is an excellent marker of thoracic situs and is of particular importance when situs ambiguus is suspected because of a central liver. When the cardiac apex is to the left, laevocardia is said to be present. Dextrocardia implies a right sided apex and the term mesocardia is used when the apex cannot be identified. When dextrocardia accompanies situs inversus, the heart is frequently normal ('mirror image' dextrocardia). Conversely, dextrocardia with situs solitus (isolated dextrocardia) strongly suggests cardiac malformations, in particular those associated with discordant atrioventricular connexions. It must be stressed that a term such as 'dextrocardia' does not describe a specific cardiac anomaly.

The most important feature of the chest X-ray in congenital heart disease is the state of the pulmonary vasculature. In the peripheral lung

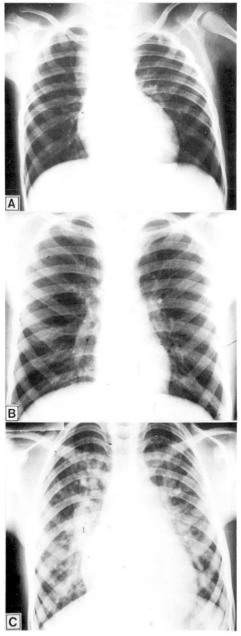

Fig. 7.1 Radiographs showing (A) pulmonary oligaemia, (B) normal pulmonary vascular markings, and (C) pulmonary plethora. Note that Fig. 7. 1(A) is from a patient with tetralogy of Fallot. A right aortic arch and pulmonary artery bay (concavity) are present.

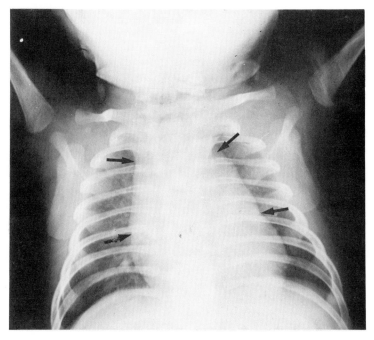

Fig. 7.2 Chest radiograph from an infant illustrating how the thymus (between arrows) gives a spurious appearance of cardiomegaly.

fields, it must always be stated whether the vascular markings are normal (Fig. 7.1B), increased (pulmonary plethora) (Fig. 7.1C), or decreased (pulmonary oligaemia) (Fig. 7.1A). It may not always be easy to make this distinction, particularly in neonates, since normality at this age resembles what might be considered as mild oligaemia in adults. In all cases, the right and left lungs should be compared with each other, as should upper and lower zones. The normal regional distribution of flow results in the lower lobe vessels appearing larger than those in the upper zone. Plethora is frequently associated with reversal of this pattern. Prominent upper lobe vessels, however, are the cardinal sign of pulmonary venous hypertension or congestion. Here a distinction must be made between an increase in size of pulmonary veins and arteries. This can be elucidated only by determining the direction of the vessels, the peripheral arteries radiating out from the main pulmonary trunk, and the veins running straight towards the left atrium. Vessels taking an abnormal direction may be bronchial arteries or systemic pulmonary collaterals, particularly in pulmonary atresia with ventricular septal defect.

The heart size and silhouette are now considered. In the first year of life cardiomegaly is definitely present if the transverse cardiothoracic ratio is 60 per cent or more. Magnification factors should be taken into account when assessing this ratio, especially if the film is taken in the antero-posterior rather than postero-anterior direction. In infants the thymus may give a spurious impression of cardiac enlargement (Fig. 7.2).

The side of the aortic arch with respect to the trachea is easily assessed on penetrated films. When a right aortic arch is found with pulmonary oligaemia (Fig. 7.1A), tetralogy of Fallot or pulmonary atresia with ventricular septal defect are likely. With plethora a right arch suggests the presence of truncus arteriosus.

Examination of the pulmonary segment gives an indication of the size of the main pulmonary artery. A concave bay indicates a small

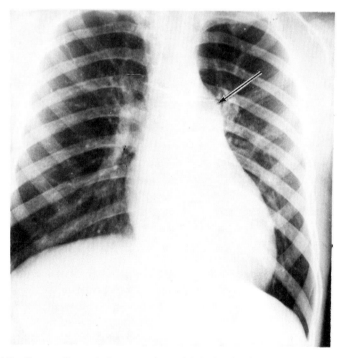

Fig. 7.3 Chest radiograph from a patient with isolated valvar pulmonary stenosis. Pulmonary vascular markings are normal but there is a prominent main pulmonary artery segment (arrowed) consequent to post-stenotic dilatation.

artery and suggests tetralogy of Fallot or pulmonary atresia with ventricular septal defect (Fig. 7.1A). A main pulmonary artery segment may also not be visible in conditions where the vessel is displaced to the right, the commonest example of which is complete transposition of the great arteries. A convex shadow would indicate a large main pulmonary artery, and if peripheral vascular markings are normal suggests pulmonary stenosis with post-stenotic dilatation (Fig. 7.3). Main pulmonary artery dilatation may be isolated, so-called idiopathic dilatation of the pulmonary artery. The main pulmonary artery is also dilated with increased pulmonary flow when peripheral vascular markings are also increased. In the hypoplastic left heart syndrome or other anomalies associated with decreased aortic flow, the main pulmonary artery will be enlarged.

Enlargement of the ascending aorta is seen in valvar aortic stenosis and is even more marked in aortic incompetence (Fig. 7.4). A straight upper left heart border may indicate an anterior left-sided ascending

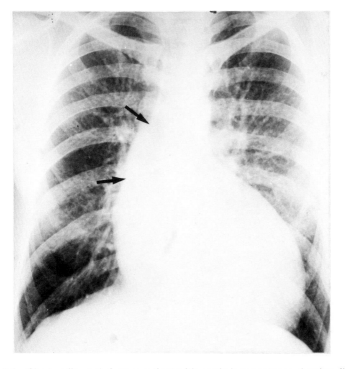

Fig. 7.4 Chest radiograph from a patient with aortic incompetence showing dilatation of the ascending aorta (between arrows).

aorta as is most commonly found in congenitally corrected transposition.

Left atrial enlargement in congenital heart disease is usually appreciated from upward displacement of the left main bronchus. This is seen in left-to-right shunts at ventricular and arterial level. Mitral valve disease, either congenital or rheumatic, also can cause marked left atrial enlargement.

References

Jefferson, K. and Rees, S. (1973). *Clinical cardiac radiology*. Butterworths, London.

Partridge, J. B., Scott, O., Deverall, P. B., and Macartney, F. J. (1975). Visualisation and measurement of the main bronchi by tomography as an objective indicator of thoracic situs in congenital heart disease. *Circulation* **51**, 188.

Van Mierop, L. H. S., Eisen, S., and Schiebler, G. L. (1970). The radiographic appearance of the tracheobronchial tree as an indicator of visceral situs. *American Journal of Cardiology* **26**, 432.

8 Investigations: the electrocardiogram

When evaluating the ECG of children with suspected congenital heart disease, it is sensible always to pose a series of specific questions. The approach should also be pragmatic and the ECG considered under two differing sets of clinical circumstances. The first instance is when an asymptomatic child is referred with a systolic murmur and the problem of presence or absence of organic cardiac disease arises. In this circumstance, the 'null hypothesis' is adopted. Wide criteria are used for normality and it is assumed that there is *no* electrocardiographic abnormality unless proved otherwise. The second situation is when a child has an overt structural cardiac anomaly. It should then be asked how the ECG can help to localize and quantitate the underlying anatomico-physiological disturbances. Inferences can be drawn from the ECG as to which ventricle is enlarged. Whether a given lesion is left- or right-sided may be evident even when absolute QRS voltage values are within normal limits.

It must be remembered that recording of lead V_4R is mandatory in all children with suspected congenital heart disease.

ECG analysis

1. *What are the rate and rhythm?* Heart-rate is less at birth than at one month, after which there is a gradual slowing with increasing age. The high rates achieved by normal infants are not always appreciated (Table 8.2). Most patients with congenital heart disease are in sinus rhythm. Paroxysmal supraventricular tachycardia may occur in otherwise normal infants. Although usually due to re-entry tachycardias, they may result from atrial fibrillation or flutter. Congenital heart block seldom causes symptoms and rarely requires specific treatment. It should be considered in any child with a resting heart-rate below the minimum for age (Table 8.1).

2. *Is there atrial hypertrophy?* Atrial hypertrophy is present when the P-wave amplitude in lead II is greater then 0.28 mV at any age. P-wave duration is seldom helpful in deciding whether right or left atrial

Table 8.1

Age	Heart rate (beats per min)				
	Min.	5%	Mean	95%	Max.
0–24 hours	85	94	119	145	145
1–7 days	100	100	133	175	175
8–30 days	115	115	163	190	190
1–3 months	115	124	154	190	205
3–6 months	115	111	140	179	205
6–12 months	115	112	140	177	175
1–3 years	100	98	126	163	190
3–5 years	55	65	98	132	145
5–8 years	70	70	96	115	145
8–12 years	55	55	79	107	115
12–16 years	55	55	75	102	115

hypertrophy is present, but prolongation to greater than 0·10 s suggests left atrial hypertrophy.

3. *Is there an abnormality of conduction?* Atrioventricular conduction is assessed by measurement of the P–R interval. This increases with age. In practice, under one year values of 0·07–0·12 s are normal. Over one year the range is 0·09–0·16 s. Shorter values suggest presence of ventricular pre-excitation and longer values indicate first-degree heart block.

The sequence of ventricular activation is principally judged from the

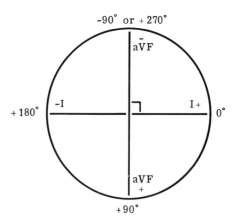

Fig. 8.1 The orientation of orthogonal leads 1 and aVF in the frontal plane. The conventions used for the calculation of mean frontal QRS axis are indicated.

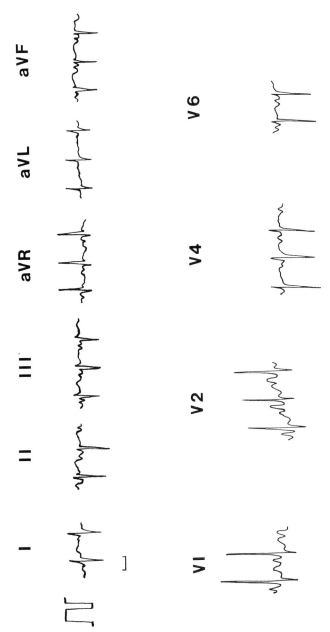

Fig. 8.2 ECG from a three month old patient with an atrioventricular canal malformation. The mean frontal QRS axis is −110° (superior axis). Note the dominantly negative forces (S wave) in aVF. There is right ventricular hypertrophy as indicated by upright T-waves and a 23 mV R-wave in V1.

Table 8.2

Age	QRS axis (frontal plane)				
	Min.	5%	Mean	95%	Max.
0–24 hours	60	60	135	180	180
1–7 days	60	80	125	160	180
8–30 days	0	60	110	160	180
1–3 months	20	40	80	120	120
3–6 months	40	20	65	80	100
6–12 months	20	0	65	100	120
1–3 years	0	20	55	100	100
3–5 years	0	40	60	80	80
5–8 years	− 20	40	65	100	100
8–12 years	0	20	65	80	120
12–16 years	− 20	20	65	80	100

mean frontal QRS axis. This is a method of summarizing one aspect of
the electrical activity of the ventricles, namely the overall direction of
electrical forces in the frontal plane. By convention, leads I, II, III,
aVR, aVL, and aVF are in the frontal plane. The axis is most simply
calculated by considering leads I and aVF. These are at right angles to
one another, i.e. orthogonal leads (Fig. 8.1). The sequence of calculation is

  a Calculate the algebraic sum of the QRS forces in leads I and aVF
    (i.e. (height of R wave) − (height of S wave));
  b Mark off each value in arbitrary units on leads I and aVF;
  c Draw lines at right angles passing through these two points;
  d A line joining the point of junction of the constructed lines to the
    point of intersect of the leads (O) is the direction of the mean
    frontal QRS vector.

Normal values are given in Table 8.2. In adults an inferior axis
greater than +110° is considered as right-axis deviation, whereas an
axis more negative than −30° is termed left-axis deviation. These
terms and values are of less help in congenital heart disease in children.
First it is more sensible to state the axis in degrees. Secondly, values of
greater than +110° can be normal for the first few years of life. The
term 'superior axis' is preferable to 'left-axis deviation' and is present
whenever QRS forces in aVF are dominantly negative. Presence of a
superior axis, especially in early infancy, strongly suggests congenital
heart disease. It is particularly associated with atrioventricular canal
defects (Fig. 8.2) and univentricular hearts with or without tricuspid
atresia (absent right atrioventricular connexion).

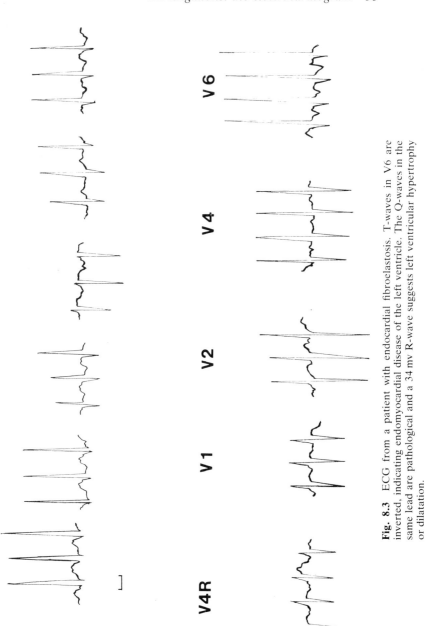

Fig. 8.3 ECG from a patient with endocardial fibroelastosis. T-waves in V6 are inverted, indicating endomyocardial disease of the left ventricle. The Q-waves in the same lead are pathological and a 34 mv R-wave suggests left ventricular hypertrophy or dilatation.

Bundle branch block can be considered to be present at any age when the QRS complex is greater than 0·10 s.

4. *Is ventricular hypertrophy present?* Hypertrophy is assessed from the R and S voltages and from the T-wave patterns in the chest leads. T-waves in V_4R and V_1 are upright at birth, but by seven days should be inverted. Failure of these right-sided T-waves to invert indicates right ventricular hypertrophy (Fig. 8.2). The T-waves stay inverted in the majority of subjects until puberty when they again become upright. T-waves in V_6 and V_7 are normally upright. Inverted left-sided T-waves indicate severe left ventricular hypertrophy or endomyocardial disease (e.g. endocardial fibroelastosis; Fig. 8.3).

QRS voltages show great variability in normal children of the same age. None the less, knowledge of normal standards is required for proper interpretation of the ECG as without voltage criteria evidence of ventricular hypertrophy will be missed. Compared with the adult, the newborn has right ventricular dominance, the RV:LV weight ratio being about 1·3:1. Changes rapidly occur so that by six months the ratio is reversed at 1:2 (compared with the adult ration of 1:2·5). This is reflected in the QRS voltages and detailed values have been

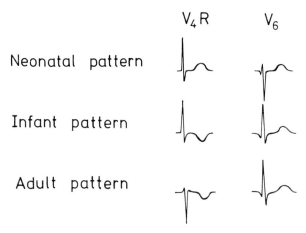

Fig. 8.4 RS progression in chest leads. The neonatal pattern of dominant R-wave in V_4R and dominant S-wave in V_6 is found in the first month of life, the infant pattern, dominant R-wave V_4R, dominant R-wave V_6, is found between one month and eighteen months and the adult pattern, dominant S-wave in V_4R, dominant R-wave in V_6, is found after this age. The presence of neonatal pattern after a month of age or infant pattern after 18 months of age indicates right ventricular hypertrophy. Conversely the presence of the adult pattern in a neonate would indicate left or posterior ventricular hypertrophy or dominance.

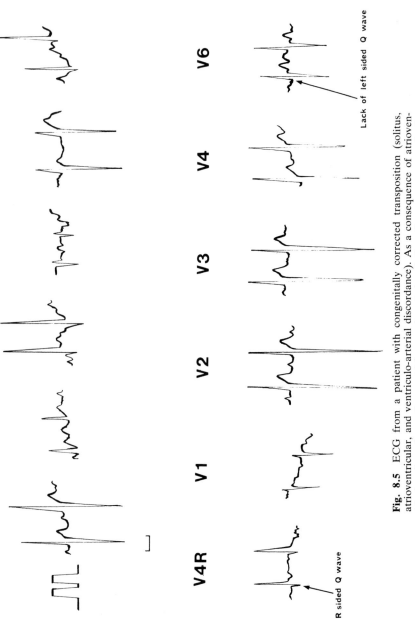

Fig. 8.5 ECG from a patient with congenitally corrected transposition (solitus, atrioventricular, and ventriculo-arterial discordance). As a consequence of atrioventricular discordance the ventricles are inverted and thus Q-waves are seen in the right-sided rather than the left-sided chest leads.

assembled by Liebman (1978). As a general rule, right ventricular hypertrophy is indicated by R-waves in $V_4R > 15$ mV under three months and > 10 mV over this age. Left ventricular hypertrophy is indicated by R waves in $V_6 > 20$ mV under three months and > 25 mV over three months. In the first month of life the R-wave is larger than the S-wave in V_4R and V_1, whereas the S-wave is larger than the R-wave in the left chest leads (sometimes called neonatal pattern) (Fig. 8.4). The 'infant' pattern is said to be present when $R > S$ in both right and left-sided chest leads, and the 'adult' pattern is when $R < S$ in V_4R, V_1 and $S > R$ in V_6 and V_7. These patterns are particularly useful in differential diagnosis of cyanotic congenital heart disease. The majority of such anomalies are characterized by right ventricular hypertrophy or right ventricular dominance (neonatal or possibly infant pattern). If the adult pattern (i.e. LV dominance) is present in an infant with cyanotic heart disease, a univentricular heart of left ventricular type with or without absent right atrioventricular connexion should be suspected. Alternatively in neonates pulmonary atresia with intact ventricular septum or critical pulmonary stenosis with small right ventricle should be considered.

The criterion for biventricular hypertrophy most commonly employed is the Katz–Wachtel phenomenon, present when R+S waves in one of the transitional leads (V_3, V_4) > 70 mV.

5. *What is the ventricular morphology?* When a ventricular septum is present, septal activation normally occurs from left to right. Q-waves are seen in leads V_6 and V_7 but not in V_4R and V_1, assuming the heart to be left-sided (i.e. levocardia). Presence of deep Q-waves in V_4R, V_1 with absent Q-waves in V_6, V_7 suggests ventricular inversion (i.e. discordant atrioventricular connexions, assuming situs solitus) (Fig. 8.5). This pattern may also be found with right ventricular hypertrophy although usually left-sided Q-waves are also present. Dominant S-waves right across the chest in leads V_4R, V_{1-6} suggest the presence of a univentricular heart.

References

Alimurung, M. M., Joseph, L. G., Nadas, A. S., and Massell, B. F. (1951). The unipolar precordial and extremely electrocardiogram in normal infants and children. *Circulation*, **4**, 420.

Liebman, J., and Plonsey, R. (1978). Electrocardiography. In *Heart disease in infants, children and adolescents* (ed. A. J. Moss, F. H. Adams, and G. C. Emmanonilides), 2nd Edn. Williams and Wilkins, Baltimore.

9 Investigations: echocardiography

Echocardiography is a means of recording the position of intracardiac surfaces using reflected ultrasound from a transducer held against the chest wall. Interest in the technique has recently increased considerably. In contrast to the discrete successive frames of an angiocardiogram in which margins are frequently ill-defined, echocardiography makes possible unequivocal demonstration of those structures whose pattern of movement is characteristic. Thus, where an angiogram may leave doubt as to the presence or position of a particular part of the heart, an echocardiogram may allow positive identification. However, failure to demonstrate a structure by echocardiography should not be taken as evidence of its absence. The technique is also attractive to those interested in cardiac function, and, because of its relative simplicity compared with other techniques and because it involves no discomfort to the patient, echocardiography may be used to make serial observations, for example, of chamber size or wall thickness. It is therefore of value in following the course of a disease or its response to treatment. The simplicity of the technique is reflected by the relatively low cost of echocardiographic systems, and this has resulted in their increasing application in areas where financial considerations are important.

The earliest and still most generally used echocardiographic method is with a single beam. The transducer is held by hand and aimed so that the beam traverses the heart. The usual ultrasound frequency is 2·25 MHz which provides excellent penetration and satisfactory resolution for most purposes. Increasing the frequency improves resolution of depth at the cost of reduced penetration, and for examining infants it is sometimes useful to use a 5 MHz transducer with a narrow beam or, exceptionally, still higher frequencies. In the so-called 'M-mode' display of the single beam technique, depth is plotted on the Y-axis against time so that to-and-fro motion along the line of the beam is represented by an oscillating line on the recording. This method provides the best resolution and clearest tracings, but is limited by the fact that only a small region of the heart is examined at any moment. This can be circumvented to some extent by moving the angle of the transducer during recording, so that the beam passes through different structures successively. The resulting 'sweep' may then be used to demonstrate the proximity of structures, and under some circumstances to determine whether or not they are in direct physical continuity with one another.

In a normal echocardiogram, chamber and vessel lumina appear as echo-free spaces. However, for demonstrating abnormal physiology, in particular intracardiac shunts, echocardiography can be considerably enhanced by the use of intravascular injections of media which reflect the echo beam, a situation directly analogous to the use of contrast material in angiography. It has been found that such reflective contrast is provided by almost any fluid immediately after injection into the circulation, because of the presence of very small bubbles. These are removed by passage through a capillary bed so that if, for example, after injection of 5 per cent dextrose into a peripheral vein echoes are obtained from blood within the left side of the heart, this implies the existence of an intracardiac right-to-left shunt. The level of shunting may be inferred from the chamber in which the bubbles first appear. This type of technique is particularly valuable when combined with intra-vascular catheterization so that injections may be given directly into particular sites.

More recently a number of instruments have been developed for two-dimensional echocardiography, in which a moving image is displayed on a television screen and recorded on videotape. The simplest involves use of an array of transducers fixed parallel to one another in a single hand-held unit. However, the method has several disadvantages which limits its clarity. In particular, the transducers pick up echoes from one another—'cross talk'—and the size of the transducer array often prevents all of it being in contact simultaneously with the chest. There is now more interest in 'sector-scanner' systems in which a sector of between 30° and 90° is scanned by a rapidly oscillating beam. This may be steered mechanically using a single vibrating transducer or electronically in a 'phased array' system. In the latter several transducers are mounted together and their combined output is used in a single wave front which is steered by staggering the order of activation of the individual crystals. Such a system has a number of theoretical advantages over the mechanical sector scanner, arising particularly from the flexibility of the electronic steering which provides an adjustable 'acoustic lens', and although it is more costly than the mechanical apparatus, this is likely to be compensated by enhanced quality of the images obtained. Single 'stopped' video frames contain only a small

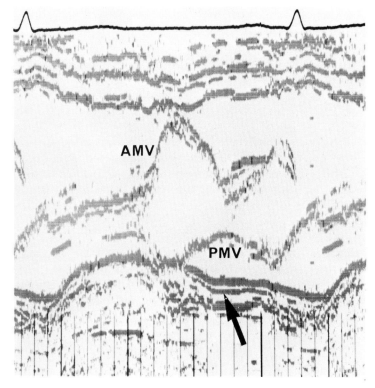

Fig. 9.1 Normal mitral echogram. AMV: anterior mitral valve leaflet. PMV: posterior leaflet. Anterior to the valve, at the top of the picture, is the septal endocardium. Posterior to the valve is the free wall (arrowed).

fraction of the information of the moving picture, and this chapter will therefore be illustrated for the most part with M-mode tracings.

The normal echocardiogram

In the normal subject it is seldom difficult to identify the mitral valve, which is characterized by the rapid forwards opening movement of its anterior cusp, followed by partial closure at the end of rapid filling and by re-opening at the time of atrial systole. The posterior cusp shows a similar pattern of diastolic movement in mirror image with lesser amplitude (Fig. 9.1). During systole the cusp echoes join, usually into a single line, and move forwards, approximately parallel to the endocardium of the posterior wall which lies behind. The free left ventricular wall thickens during systole, and becomes thinner during early diastole. Anterior to the mitral valve is the interventricular septum. The left side usually moves posteriorly during systole and then forwards during left ventricular filling, so that the diameter of the left ventricle, measured between the endocardial surfaces of the septum and posterior wall, lessens throughout systole and increases, at first rapidly and then more slowly, during diastole. Anterior to the interventricular septum lies the right ventricular cavity. Its dimension is more variable than that of the left ventricle, since small variations in the position of the transducer may cause the beam to transect widely different diameters. The tricuspid valve leaflets may appear on the same recording as the mitral valve, but are often best shown with the transducer aimed more medially. The anterior tricuspid leaflet has a similar pattern of movement to that of the mitral valve, but its septal leaflet has a restricted range of movement because its base is completely attached to the septum (Fig. 9.2).

Angling the ultrasound beam upwards and medial from the position in which it traverses the ventricles and mitral valve causes it to pass through the posterior great artery, and left atrium. The aortic root reflects two echoes moving to and fro in parallel with between them the right and posterior aortic valve cusps opening and closing. On an

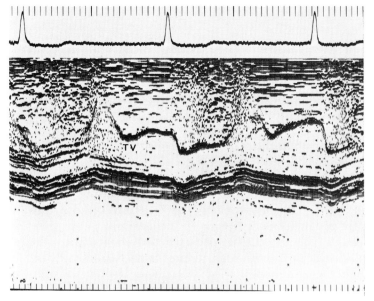

Fig. 9.2 Normal tricuspid valve echogram. TV: tricuspid valve.

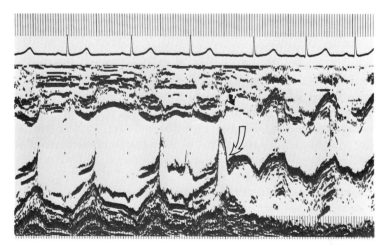

Fig. 9.3 Normal subject: sweep from left ventricular cavity at the left side through the level of the mitral valve to the aortic root and left atrium. Note continuity between the anterior wall of the aorta and septum and the posterior wall of aorta and anterior mitral leaflet (arrow).

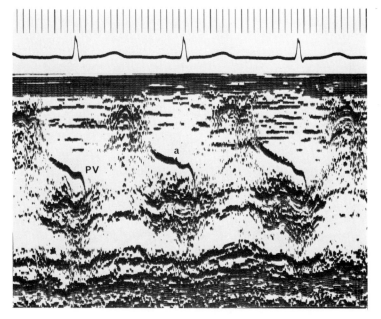

Fig. 9.4 Normal pulmonary valve (PV) echogram. Only one leaflet is identifiable. Before its rapid posterior opening movement, there is a typical 'A' wave (a).

M-mode 'sweep' (Fig. 9.3), or a longitudinal section made with the sector scanner it is possible to demonstrate the normal continuity of the posterior aortic root with the anterior leaflet of the mitral valve and of the anterior part of the aorta with the interventricular septum. Anterior to the aortic valve lies the right ventricular outflow tract. In many subjects it is possible to identify a cusp of the pulmonary valve above and to the left of the aortic valve. This shows not only a posterior opening movement at the onset of systole followed by closure similar to the posterior aortic valve cusp, but also a brief and smaller displacement corresponding to atrial systole (Fig. 9.4).

The ventricles and interventricular septum
The echocardiographer is frequently called upon to determine whether or not there is an inlet ventricular septum dividing the atrioventricular valves. In order to demonstrate the presence of this structure, it is necessary to show its double-sidedness by finding echoes from both right and left ventricular endocardium. Having defined the position of the septum, it is possible to estimate the absolute and relative sizes of

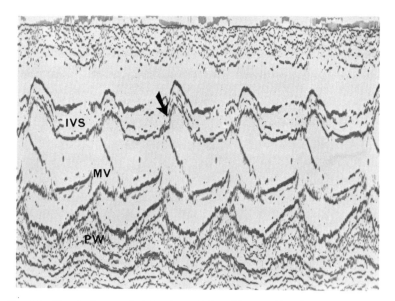

Fig. 9.5   Ventricular septal defect in an infant. Note rapid wall movement at the onset of filling with very fast anterior movement of the septum (IVS) (arrowed). MV: mitral valve. PW: posterior left ventricular wall.

the ventricular cavities. Dilatation of the left ventricle in both systole and diastole, with reduced wall excursion, can readily be demonstrated in patients with myocardial disease, for example in cardiomyopathy, endocardial fibroelastosis, or infarction. This should be contrasted with increased end-diastolic dimension but normal or reduced end-systolic dimension which indicates increased left ventricular stroke volume as in aortic regurgitation, mitral regurgitation, or ventricular septal defect. In the last two conditions, rapid adoption by the cavity of a spherical configuration at the onset of filling is manifest as fast separation of the septal and posterior wall endocardium, often with a striking anterior movement of the septum (Fig. 9.5). Reduction in left ventricular cavity size may be associated with left ventricular hypertrophy or inflow obstruction. In the former, hypertrophy affects both the free wall and septum, not always to the same degree so that their relative dimensions may vary. Thus no particular significance should be attached to apparently disproportionate septal hypertrophy. Hypertrophic cardiomyopathy, which may be primary or secondary, is characterized not only by a small cavity size and wall hypertrophy, but also by various abnormalities of relaxation.

In the newborn, severe reduction in left ventricular cavity size, so that its end-diastolic dimension is less than 1 cm, associated with reduced amplitude of the mitral valve echogram and absent aortic cusp

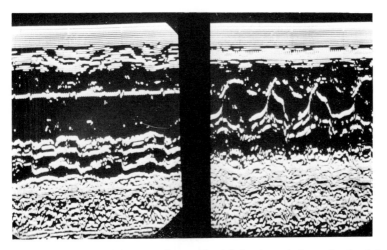

Fig. 9.6 Hypoplastic left heart syndrome. The left hand panel shows the tiny left ventricular cavity with minimal excursion of the mitral valve. On the right is the large right ventricle containing the tricuspid valve echogram.

echoes (Fig. 9.6), indicate the hypoplastic left heart syndrome. These appearances are often sufficiently characteristic to obviate the need for cardiac catheterization.

Even in the neonate the transverse right ventricular dimension is normally less than the left ventricular diameter. Enlargement or relative preponderance of the right ventricular cavity usually indicates a left-to-right shunt at atrial level. In atrial septal defect, when uncomplicated by a left-sided lesion, right ventricular overload is also indicated by reversal of septal movement, in that at the level of the echobeam the septum moves in a posterior direction during filling and forwards during systole (Fig. 9.7). The right ventricular cavity may also

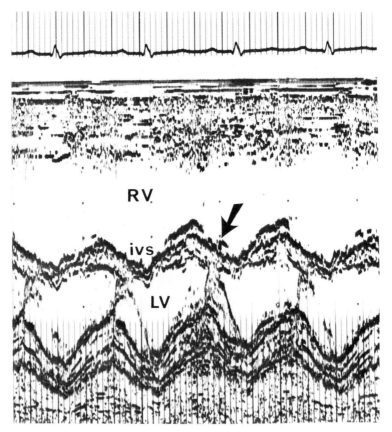

Fig. 9.7   Secundum atrial septal defect. The right ventricular cavity is large. Movement of the septum (ivs) is reversed (arrow).

be enlarged in conditions causing a high right ventricular pressure, even with a normal flow, particularly transposition of the great arteries.

Failure to record a septal echogram may be because this structure is abnormally oriented, for example in congenitally corrected transposition. The diagnosis of univentricular heart by M-mode requires not only absence of septal echoes, but also other characteristic and positive findings. The diagnosis is most easily made where there are two inlet valves because in these patients the two medial atrioventricular valve leaflets—the posterior leaflet of the right valve and the anterior leaflet of the left valve—appear to touch or overlap at the beginning of diastole (Fig. 9.8). This occurs not only because there are no interposed echoes from the septum, but also by virtue of the increased mobility of the 'septal' leaflet of the anterior valve resulting from absence of its normal attachment, this alone being a useful characteristic. Thus even when the posterior atrioventricular valve is

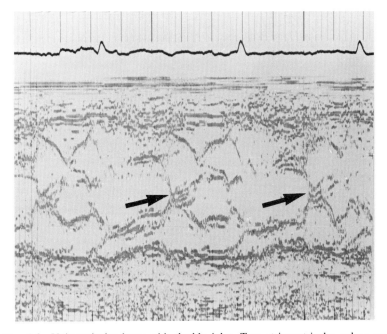

Fig. 9.8 Univentricular heart with double inlet. Two atrioventricular valves are clearly seen. The posterior leaflet of the anterior valve shows abnormally wide excursion and appears to touch the posterior valve during early diastole. No septum can be seen (arrows).

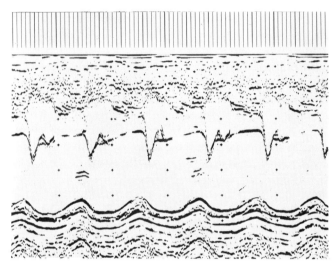

Fig. 9.9 Univentricular heart with absent left atrioventricular connexion. Only one ventricular cavity could be identified. The atrioventricular valve lies anterior and its posterior leaflet shows the typical wide excursion seen with absence of the posterior septum.

absent or dysplastic, the diagnosis may still be made from the morphology of the anterior inlet valve, for besides often being large it exhibits, as in double inlet, the typical wide excursion of its large unsupported posterior leaflet (Fig. 9.9). In cases of absent right atrioventricular connexion including 'tricuspid atresia' typically the posterior (mitral) valve is large and lies somewhat anteriorly. Its posterior cusp is large, so that the movements of the valve appear almost symmetrical (Fig. 9.10). In some cases the appearances of the valve and sub-valve apparatus may be confusing, even resembling two distinct valves, and it is not always possible to make a definite echocardiographic diagnosis.

In many cases of univentricular heart it is possible to demonstrate an anterior septum separating a rudimentary outlet chamber from the main chamber. This, of course, cannot contain an inlet valve, but may be shown to support a great artery. Distinction between left ventricular and right ventricular types of univentricular heart is not usually possible, since from the functional standpoint they behave similarly. However, the rare finding of a posterior rudimentary chamber is highly

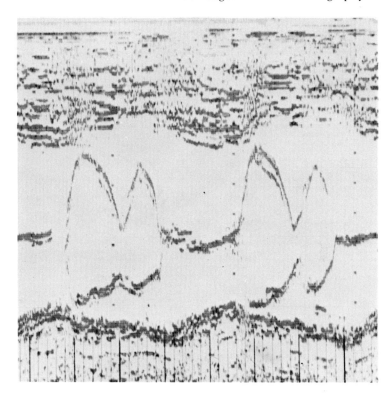

Fig. 9.10 Absent right atrioventricular connexion (tricuspid atresia). Typical appearance of the single atrioventricular valve in a ten-year-old patient. Note the anterior position of the valve with large posterior leaflet.

suggestive that the anterior main chamber is of right ventricular type (Fig. 9.11).

It is not possible to demonstrate ventricular septal defects by M-mode echocardiography, except where there is over-ride of a great artery, or by inference from the left ventricular filling pattern. The appearances described for univentricular heart are not seen in large septal defects.

The valves
The atrioventricular valve echograms are easy to identify and frequently yield diagnostic information. In mitral stenosis, whether congenital or acquired, the normal rapid early diastolic valve closure is absent. Instead, the anterior cusp, having opened fully, moves slowly backwards throughout diastole, before closing at the onset of systole.

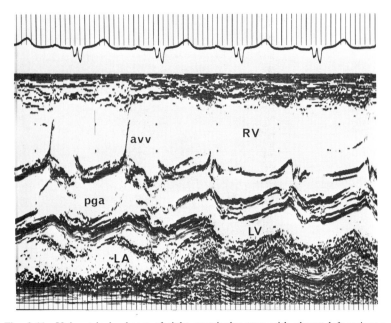

Fig. 9.11 Univentricular heart of right ventricular type with absent left atrioventricular connexion. A single valve (avv) is seen, lying within the right ventricular cavity "RV". There is a posterior septum with behind it a rudimentary chamber of left ventricular type "LV". The latter communicates with but does not support half of the posterior great artery (pga). There is no communication between left atrium (LA) and the posterior chamber.

The posterior cusp behaves in a similar fashion and, because of commissural fusion, its opening movement is forwards in the same direction as that of the anterior cusp. In congenital mitral stenosis the cusps are thin and appear so on the echogram, whereas rheumatic thickening of the cusp causes multiple echoes from both (Fig. 9.12). Reduction in amplitude of anterior cusp movement is a feature of severe rheumatic disease and results from shrinkage and stiffening of the sub-valve apparatus. It is not possible reliably to estimate the degree of inflow obstruction solely from the appearance of the mitral valve echogram. The 'diastolic closure rate' of the anterior cusp gives only a very approximate guide. However, disturbance of the left ventricular filling pattern may be inferred from the pattern of wall movement during diastole. Slow and protracted filling is shown by slow and progressive increase in cavity dimension throughout diastole, often associated with reversal of septal movement. The same signs of slow left ventricular filling are seen with other causes of left ventricular inflow obstruction,

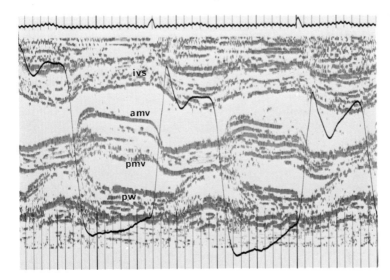

Fig. 9.12 Severe rheumatic mitral stenosis. The mitral valve cusps reflect multiple echoes and the diastolic closure rate is reduced. Overall amplitude of opening is reduced and the posterior cusp moves forwards in diastole. The left ventricular cavity size is normal. Note that there is continuous slow separation of the walls throughout diastole. The superimposed tracing is the apex cardiogram.

of which the most important in paediatric practice are cor triatriatum and patch obstruction after Mustard's operation for complete transposition of the great arteries. In the case of cor triatriatum, it may be possible to demonstrate the abnormal membrane lying within the left atrial cavity behind the aortic root. That the abnormal echo is not simply an additional aortic root echo is shown by the variable distance between it and the posterior part of the aorta.

Non-rheumatic mitral regurgitation is not usually accompanied by diagnostic changes in the valve echogram. Rather, its severity may be inferred from the rapidity of increase in left ventricular dimension in early diastole, as in ventricular septal defect. Systolic prolapse, which is usually associated with mild regurgitation, may be demonstrable as transient backward displacement of one or other mitral valve leaflet during late or sometimes all of systole (Fig. 9.13). This movement is often synchronous with a systolic click.

The most important congenital lesion affecting the tricuspid valve is Ebstein's anomaly. Here, the echocardiographic features are as variable as is the pathological severity. In forms of clinical importance,

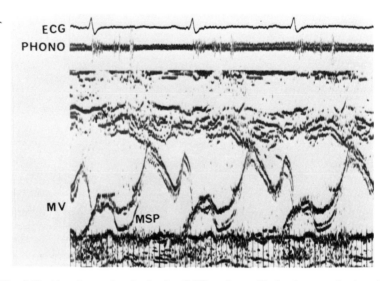

Fig. 9.13 Non-rheumatic mitral valve (MV) prolapse. During late systole there is pronounced posterior displacement of part of the anterior mitral valve leaflet (MSP). This is associated with two systolic clicks recorded on the phonocardiogram (PHONO).

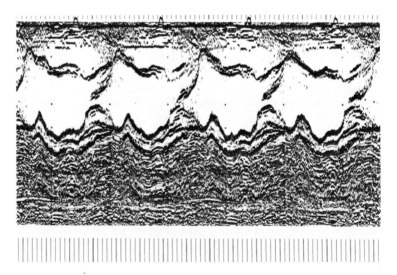

Fig. 9.14 Ebstein's anomaly: the tricuspid valve is large, and the leaflets exhibit abnormally wide movements.

however, it is usual to find conspicuous wide excursion of the anterior tricuspid leaflet which appears to occupy a dilated right ventricular cavity (Fig. 9.14). The disorder of interventricular conduction which frequently accompanies this condition manifests itself by asynchrony of closure of the two atrioventricular valves.

Echocardiography may contribute to accurate diagnosis of atrioventricular canal defects, since it is usually possible in the complete form to demonstrate the existence of a common atrioventricular valve leaflet. Although 'mitral' and 'tricuspid' valves may be shown separately with certain positions of the transducer, there is usually a position in which the common anterior leaflet, straddling the top of the interventricular septum as it does, appears to pass through it on the echo (Fig. 9.15). In partial canal defects, this is usually not the case, and the only clue, for example in a primum atrial septal defect, may be evidence of abnormal insertion of the mitral valve, revealed in the way that it lies abnormally anterior, close to the interventricular septum, and moves parallel to it during diastole (Fig. 9. 16). If there is significant left-to-right shunting, then septal movement is usually reversed and the right ventricle dilated. By contrast, rapid left ventricular filling may indicate mitral regurgitation. Cine angiograms in these conditions are often difficult to interpret and the echocardiogram, using either M-mode or two-dimensional techniques, may facilitate precise pre-operative diagnosis,

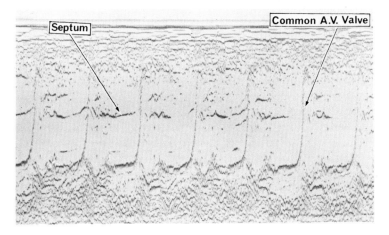

Fig. 9.15 Complete atrioventricular canal showing the classical appearance of the anterior common leaflet appearing to pass through the interventricular septum.

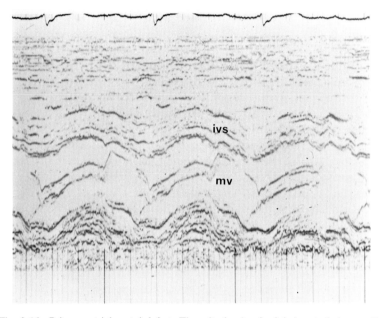

Fig. 9.16   Primum atrial septal defect. The mitral valve (mv) is inserted abnormally anterior, lying approximately in the middle of the left ventricular cavity during systole. The diastolic movements of the anterior leaflet closely parallel the septum (ivs), the motion of which is reversed.

particularly with regard to cusp anatomy and the sub-valve attachments.

Congenital disease of the aortic valve is often not apparent on M-mode echocardiography. When the valve is bicuspid, asymmetrical closing of the cusps within the aorta may indicate the diagnosis, but specificity of this finding is unproven, and in a number of cases it does not occur.

Murmurs arising in the ventricular outflow tracts are associated with prominent vibration of the cusps of the arterial valves. In sub-valvar obstruction this vibration is coarsened so that the cusps move briefly almost to their closed position in early systole. In valvar pulmonary stenosis, the movement of the posterior cusp provides some insight into the pattern of pulmonary artery flow, for the A wave of the cusp is frequently accentuated to the extent that the valve appears to open with atrial systole and remain partially open until ventricular systole. This is consistent with the frequent finding that the right ventricular end diastolic pressure exceeds the pulmonary artery diastolic pressure.

Overriding great arteries and abnormal connexions

There are a number of conditions in which abnormal spatial relationships, in particular those affecting the root of the posterior great artery,
may be demonstrated by an M-mode sweep. When there is aortic
override, as in Fallot's tetralogy, it is frequently possible to show that
the anterior wall of the aortic root lies appreciably anterior to the top of
the septum, while the posterior part remains continuous with the
anterior mitral valve cusp (Fig. 9. 17). While these findings may be

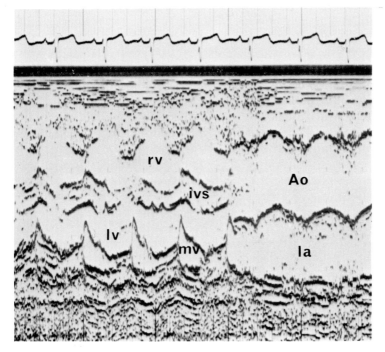

Fig. 9.17 Tetralogy of Fallot. Sweep from the ventricular cavities at the left of the
picture to aortic root and left atrium at the right. Note that the anterior wall of the
aorta lies considerably anterior to the interventricular septum. There is continuity
between mitral valve and the posterior wall of the aorta.

diagnostic, failure to demonstrate discontinuity between the septum
and the aorta should not be taken to exclude the diagnosis since the
finding probably depends upon the angle at which it is possible to make
a sweep. At some angles of the beam, just as in certain angiographic
projections, the apparent override may be minimized. The same
applies to the use of two-dimensional scanning in this context, and to

the case of double outlet right ventricle where it is again not always possible to show that more than 50 per cent of the posterior great artery lies anterior to the septum. Furthermore, discontinuity between posterior wall of the aorta and anterior mitral valve cusp, often associated with double outlet right ventricle, may not be demonstrated. In this case, the two structures are separated by fibrous tissue which, at a particular angle of the transducer, may cause apparent 'echocardiographic' continuity between the two. Override of the septum by a persistent truncus arteriosus leads to a similar echocardiographic appearance to that of tetralogy. Distinction between these two conditions is usually obvious clinically. If not, then finding an anterior arterial valve clarifies the situation. In all of these conditions, it may be possible to make a definite diagnosis by echocardiography, but it is seldom safe to exclude a diagnosis on the basis of negative findings. Congenitally corrected transposition (discordant atrioventricular and ventriculo-arterial connexions) is also associated with abnormal positions and relations of intra-cardiac structures. The septum tends to lie in a near sagittal plane, so that it is difficult to record simultaneously with the atrioventricular valves or other walls of the heart, or even sometimes to identify it at all. The right-sided mitral valve (in levocardia) is usually anterior and is distinguished from a normal tricuspid valve by the excessive amplitude of movement of its posterior cusp, similar to that seen in the univentricular heart. It may appear continuous with the posterior great artery, whereas the posterior atrioventricular valve is not continuous with the posterior part of the aorta. These findings are however variable, and in this condition it may frequently not be possible to say more than that the intra-cardiac connexions are abnormal. Use of a two-dimensional system in this context may be of value, in particular by confirming the presence of an interventricular septum, but the problem remains of identifying which inlet valve is which.

The arterial valves cannot be distinguished from one another echocardiographically either by M-mode or sector scan, so that diagnosis of abnormal ventriculo-arterial connexions or abnormal relations between the great arteries, is not straightforward. In the case of single beam echocardiography, the most useful approach has been to combine the 'contrast' technique with echocardiography from the suprasternal notch. The rationale is that whatever the position of the semilunar valves and roots of the great arteries, the arch of the aorta always lies antero-superior to the pulmonary artery, so that seen from above the sternum it necessarily appears as anterior. Having excluded right-to-left shunting at atrial or ventricular level, the diagnosis of discordant ventriculo-arterial connexions is made when reflective fluid injected into a peripheral vein appears exclusively or first in the aorta as identified from the suprasternal notch. The same approach may be used with the two-dimensional techniques, or it may often be possible to show, from the anterior chest wall, that the great artery which arises posteriorly is the pulmonary artery, by virtue of the fact that it bends posteriorly below the arch of the aorta.

References

Anderson, R. H. (1978). Cardiac anatomy. In *A programme of echocardiography* (ed. G. Leach and G. C. Sutton). Medicine, London.

Assad-Morell, J. L., Tajik, A. J., and Giuloani, E. R. (1974). Echocardiographic analysis of the ventricular septum. *Progress in Cardiovascular Disease* **17**, 219.

Feigenbaum, H. (1976). *Echocardiography*, 2nd edn. Lea & Febiger, Philadelphia.

Goldberg, S. J., Allen, H. D., and Sahn, D. J. (1975). *Paediatric and adolescent echocardiography.* Yearbook Medical Publishers, Inc., Chicago.

Meyer, R. A. (1978). Echocardiography In *Heart disease in infants, children and adolescents* (ed. A. J. Moss, F. H. Adams, and G. C. Emmanouilides), pp. 85–107. Williams & Wilkins, Baltimore.

Seward, J. B., Tajik, A. J., Spangler, J. G., and Ritter, D. G. (1975). Echocardiographic contrast studies: Initial experience. *Mayo Clinic Proceedings* **50**, 163.

10 Investigations: cardiac catheterization and angiography

Cardiac catheterization is an essential technique in the evaluation of congenital heart disease. It involves passage of a flexible catheter into the heart via a vein (right heart catheterization) and sometimes via an artery (retrograde arterial catheterization). Especially when right heart catheterization is carried out from the saphenous or femoral vein the catheter may be passed across a patent foramen ovale or atrial septal defect into the left side of the heart. Trans-septal catheterization is rarely required in the investigation of congenital heart disease. Direct left ventricular or pulmonary arterial puncture (Radner needle) are sometimes employed. The hazards of catheterization are small in major cardiac centres except for infants, who should only be investigated in centres designated for paediatric cardiology.

At catheterization, pressures and oxygen saturation should always, if possible, be measured in systemic and pulmonary veins, both atria,

Table 10.1

Q_p (l/min/m²)	=	$\dfrac{O_2 \text{ consumption ml/min/m}^2}{O_2 \text{ content (PV PA) ml/l}}$
Q_s (l/min/m²)	=	$\dfrac{O_2 \text{ consumption ml/min/m}^2}{O_2 \text{ content (Ao-SVC) ml/l}}$
Effective Q_p (l/min/m²)	=	$\dfrac{O_2 \text{ consumption ml/min/m}^2}{O_2 \text{ content (PV-SVC) ml/l}}$
Left-to-right shunt	=	Q_p – effective Q_p
Right-to-left shunt	=	Q_s – effective Q_p

Q_p = pulmonary flow; Q_s = systemic flow; PV = pulmonary vein; PA = pulmonary artery; Ao = aorta; SVC = superior vena cava.

It is apparent that if there are no shunts the O_2 content of the blood in PV is similar to that in Ao and that in the SVC is similar to that in the pulmonary artery (= mixed venous). Under these circumstances $Q_p = Q_s$ = effective Q_p. O_2 content includes dissolved O_2 as well as that bound to circulating haemoglobin. 1 g Hb combines with 1·38 ml O_2 (at S.T.P.) when fully saturated. 0·003 ml O_2 per 100 ml blood are dissolved for 1mm Hg Po_2.

Table 10.2

Pulmonary vascular resistance (PVR)	$= \dfrac{\text{Mean PA} - \text{mean LA}^* \text{ pressure (mm Hg)}}{Q_p \ (1/\text{min}/\text{m}^2)}$
Systemic vascular resistance (SVR)	$= \dfrac{\text{Mean Ao} - \text{mean RA pressure (mm Hg)}}{Q_s \ (1/\text{min}/\text{m}^2)}$

* If LA pressure cannot be measured directly then the mean pulmonary artery wedge pressure is used.

both ventricles, aorta, and pulmonary artery. There is no place for an incomplete study in the investigation of congenital heart disease.

From oxygen saturation data obtained at catheterization, pulmonary, systemic, and effective pulmonary blood flow can be calculated (Table 10.1). From these calculations the degree of left-to-right, right-to-left, or bidirectional shunting is determined. The pulmonary and systemic vascular resistances can also be calculated knowing the flows and mean pressure differences across the relevant vascular beds (Table 10. 2). To interpret the significance of an elevated pulmonary vascular resistance, however, it is critical to know the values of arterial blood gases at the time of study (see p. 36).

Flows are normally calculated using the Fick principle, from oxygen contents† of blood samples from systemic and pulmonary veins, aorta and pulmonary artery, and from the oxygen consumption per minute. The latter is often derived from tables, but is better measured directly. The concept of effective pulmonary flow allows calculation of bidirectional shunts. Effective flow is that amount of the systemic venous return that is fully oxygenated by passage through the lungs. The calculated resistances (Table 10.2) represent the ratio of pressure drop across the lungs to flow through them.

A distinction must be made between pulmonary hypertension, an elevated pulmonary vascular resistance, and pulmonary vascular disease. Pulmonary hypertension implies only that the pulmonary artery pressure is higher than expected for the age of the patient. The high blood pressure may result from an increased pulmonary blood flow, an increased pulmonary vascular resistance, or from an increased pulmo-

†With the patient breathing room air, dissolved oxygen is in practice seldom included in the calculations of flows which are usually based on oxygen contents derived from oxygen saturation data alone (i.e. Hb concentration $\times$ 1·38 $\times$ percentage of total Hb as Hbo_2, measured using oximetry). In patients breathing pure oxygen, important amounts of oxygen are transported dissolved in plasma and for accurate calculations of flows the Po_2 of the blood sample must be known to derive the true oxygen content (o_2 transported as Hbo_2 + dissolved o_2).

nary venous (wedge) pressure, as could be found in mitral stenosis or in left heart failure where the left ventricular end diastolic pressure is elevated. Elevation of pulmonary vascular resistance may be due either to pulmonary vasoconstriction (e.g. secondary to hypoxia, acidosis (low pH) or to hypoventilation (high P_{CO_2})) when it is reversible, or to pulmonary vascular disease when it is irreversible. The latter implies permanent damage to the small pulmonary arteries with endothelial proliferation, fibrosis, fibrinoid necrosis, and round-cell infiltration. When an elevated pulmonary vascular resistance is discovered it is essential to investigate its potential reversibility by administration of 100 per cent oxygen for at least five minutes. A fall under such conditions would indicate that a patient erroneously deemed inoperable because of 'pulmonary vascular disease' may be potentially suitable for corrective surgery, whereas an irreversibly

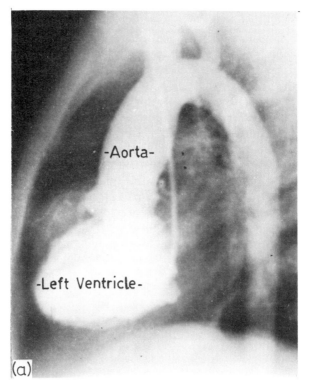

Fig. 10.1　(a) Conventional lateral left ventriculogram. (b) Angiogram performed in 'long axial view' which opens out the anterior portion of the interventricular septum and allows a very small muscular defect to be visualized (arrowed).

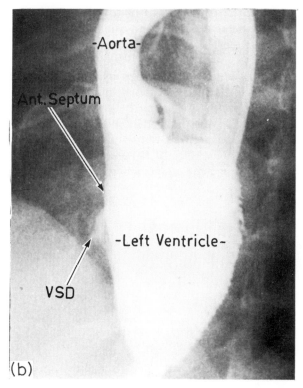

-Aorta-

Ant. Septum

-Left Ventricle-

VSD

(b)

elevated pulmonary vascular resistance would confirm inoperability.

Angiography
Angiograms would normally be performed in both ventricles and the aorta (the latter at least to exclude a persistent ductus arteriosus) unless there were firm indications to the contrary. Atrial injections are also sometimes required for the complete evaluation of complex anomalies. The study should not be considered complete unless a full segmental diagnosis of the heart under investigation has been established.

Details of angiographic techniques are beyond the scope of this book, although some of the principles may be of interest. Contrast media are iodine-containing relatively viscous fluids with a variable but usually low sodium content (Triosil is used at the Brompton Hospital). The maximum dose per injection is 2 ml/kg body weight although 1 ml/kg may be adequate. A total dosage of 4 ml/kg for all angiograms is safe although 3 ml/kg is preferable. Some centres will use more than 4 ml/kg, accepting the definite risks of so doing. Biplane cineangiography is the optimal technique and a biplane video facility which allows immediate recall of the angiogram greatly facilitates the investigation.

In complex anomalies, ventriculograms are usually performed in antero-posterior and lateral projections simultaneously. Angled views often allow better profiling and hence better definition of intra-cardiac structures, especially interatrial and interventricular septa. In acyanotic heart disease, particularly if a ventricular septal defect is suspected, the use of the long axial (Fig. 10.1b) and four-chamber views introduced by Bargeron and co-workers allows accurate anatomical siting

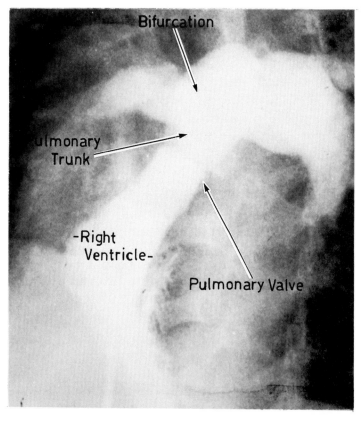

Fig. 10.2   Right ventriculogram in left anterior oblique projection with cranio-caudal tilt allowing visualization of the right ventricular outflow tract and branching of main pulmonary artery.

of the defect. Similarly, the addition of a cranio-caudal tilt to the right ventriculogram either in the frontal or left anterior oblique projection (Fig. 10.2) allows better visualization of the right ventricular outflow tract and branching of the main pulmonary artery.

References

Bargeron, L. M., Elliot, L. P., and Soto, B. (1977). Axial angiography in congenital heart disease, technical and anatomical considerations. *Circulation* **56**, 1075.

Grossman, W. (1974). *Cardiac catheterization and angiography*. Lea & Febiger, Philadelphia.

Jarmakani, J. M. (1978). Cardiac catheterization. In *Heart disease in infants, children and adolescents* (ed. A. J. Moss, F. H. Adams and G. C. Emmanouilides), pp. 107–26. Williams & Wilkins, Baltimore.

11 The principles of surgical treatment of congenital heart disease

Although historical considerations might be considered out of place in a book such as this, it is salutary to realize that open heart surgery has been possible for less than 25 years.

Surgical closure of a persistent ductus arteriosus was first suggested in 1907 by Munro, following his demonstration in 1888 that such a structure could easily be closed by ligation in an infant cadaver.

It was not until 1937 that Strieder made the first surgical attempt to close a persistent ductus arteriosus, and Gross in 1938 successfully closed a ductus in a seven-year-old girl, commencing the era of modern cardiac surgery in the treatment of congenital heart disease. Two decades passed before this structure was closed in an infant.

Following the treatment of persistent ductus arteriosus, Crafoord in 1944 successfully resected a coarctation of the aorta, and Kirklin in 1952 performed a similar operation in a ten-week-old infant. Palliative treatment of cyanotic congenital heart disease opened with the introduction of a subclavian artery/pulmonary artery anastomosis, as suggested and performed by Blalock in 1944. The operation revolutionized the treatment of patients with decreased pulmonary blood flow. It was not until 1951 that the concept of constricting (banding) the pulmonary artery to decrease pulmonary flow in patients with large left-to-right shunts was used as suggested by Muller and Dammann.

The application by Gibbon of a mechanical heart and lung apparatus to provide an extra-corporeal circuit for cardiac surgery in 1954 heralded the era of corrective intracardiac surgery, following which, at the present time, there are few congenital heart defects, either complex or simple, which cannot be now corrected—at least in the short term.

Current concepts
Patients with congenital heart disease can either undergo correction of their congenital anomaly, or a palliative operation can be performed with a view to total correction in the future.

Simple defects, such as persistent ductus arteriosus and coarctation of the aorta, can be totally corrected in infancy and early childhood. Complete intracardiac correction of congenital heart defects in early infancy may not always be possible because of the size of the patient, or the complexity of the lesion.

There are compelling sociological, psychological, economic, and surgical arguments for one-stage total correction of simple and complex congenital heart disease when the patient first requires surgical help. However, if such a policy is to be pursued, one-stage total correction must have a morbidity and mortality which is equal to or less than that from palliation followed by correction at a later date.

With ever-increasing improvement of surgical and anaesthetic techniques, together with a better understanding of myocardial and whole body preservation, there has been a move in the last ten years towards early one-stage total correction with an acceptable mortality and morbidity in many instances.

Principles of cardiopulmonary bypass for surgery of congenital heart disease

Success in the surgery of congenital heart disease is dependent upon accurate pre-operative diagnosis, perfect operative conditions, preservation of the myocardium and all the vital organs, and maintenance of total body function in the post-operative period.

Certain anomalies such as coarctation of the aorta or persistent ductus arteriosus can be treated surgically without resorting to the use of cardiopulmonary bypass machinery, since the anomaly lies outside the main chambers of the heart and does not require interruption of blood flow to the vital structures.

In order to carry out corrective surgery within the heart, cardiopulmonary bypass must be used. This entails using apparatus by which the pumping action of the heart and gas transfer of the lungs is substituted by mechanical, artificial, and physiological devices. By means of this apparatus it is possible to exclude the heart from the body, allowing intracardiac surgery to be performed. The obvious limitations of such apparatus is that the pump (artificial heart) is usually non-pulsatile, and the artificial lung is usually of the type which allows blood and gas to mix, thereby causing damage to the blood constituents. A more recent development of pulsatile pumps and membrane oxygenators has allowed great improvement in the application of cardiopulmonary bypass techniques. The addition of hypothermia, haemodilution, and isolated cardiac ischaemia using cardioplegic drugs facilitates cardiopulmonary techniques, reduces the time on the bypass machine, and thereby reduces the morbidity which can accrue from the intervention of extra-corporeal circuitry.

Hypothermia reduces oxygen consumption and metabolism thereby aiding the survival of tissue during the period of cardiopulmonary bypass perfusion.

In 'profound' hypothermia the body is cooled to 15 °C on cardiopulmonary bypass, and with moderate hypothermia to 28 °C.

In patients below the weight of 5 kg, previous surface cooling by ice-bags applied to the surface of the body reduces the patient's body temperature to 28 °C (Fig. 11.1). This has the advantage of slowing

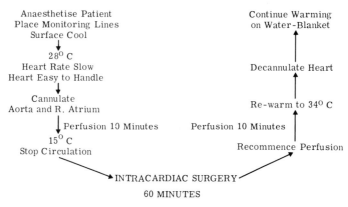

Fig. 11.1   Flow plan for treatment of surface induced hypothermia with limited cardio-pulmonary bypass.

the heart rate, and facilitates the surgery required to connect the heart to the cardiopulmonary bypass perfusion apparatus. In addition, the previous surface cooling reduces the time spent on bypass to achieve the cooling, be it moderate or profound hypothermia.

At 15 °C the circulation can be arrested for an arbitrary period of sixty minutes, during which intracardiac surgery can be performed. This gives an ideal operating field, and is particularly applicable to patients under the weight of 5 kg.

Preservation of the myocardium with good long-term function must be achieved in addition to the preservation of all other vital organs. Use of hypothermic biochemical perfusates within the coronary artery circulation and topically applied hypothermic solutions to the surface of the heart has improved the preservation of the myocardium. Immediately satisfactory cardiac function does not necessarily mean that there will be good long-term cardiac function.

Monitoring of brain activity is an important part of the overall monitoring carried out during cardiac surgery, particularly when hypothermic techniques are used (Fig. 11.2).

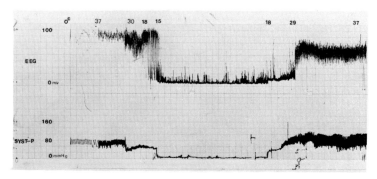

Fig. 11.2 Recordings taken during an operation showing the variation in cerebral function (upper trace EEG) and arterial blood pressure (lower trace SYST-P) during an operation. The variation in temperature is shown along the upper line in degrees Celsius. There is an alteration of cerebral function at 30 °C coincident with institution of cardio-pulmonary bypass when the systemic arterial trace becomes non-pulsatile. At 15° C cardio-pulmonary bypass is discontinued. Thereafter follows a period of circulatory arrest for 60 min and then the re-institution of cardio-pulmonary bypass at 18 °C. Pulsatile flow recommences at 29 °C with return of the cerebral function monitor record.

Monitoring during and after cardiac surgery

Since the circulation is being manipulated artificially during the period of cardiopulmonary bypass perfusion, it is important to be able to monitor certain physiological variables, in particular the central venous (right atrial) and left atrial pressures, as well as systemic arterial pressure and urine output. Frequent estimations of acid-base status and oxygenation must be performed. Cardiac rhythm is monitored by means of electrocardiogram, and during hypothermia rectal and naso-pharyngeal temperatures must be known.

Following cardiac surgery, all patients should be returned to an intensive care unit, staffed with doctors and nurses especially trained in this area of care. In the postoperative period physiological variables are monitored as during surgery. These are recorded every fifteen minutes. Blood loss via the chest drains is measured and replaced accordingly. The routine measurement of cardiac output in the postoperative period, although ideal, is not widely practised, nor in the majority of patients is this complex form of monitoring of cardiac action necessary.

Management and ventilation

It is customary for most patients to return to the intensive care unit ventilated and sedated. During the transition from the operation room to the intensive care unit it is vital that the patient is sedated, and that there is control over the airway.

In children under the age of five years a naso-endotracheal tube is preferable to an oral endotracheal tube. The former is more easily held in place, and may be required for several days (Fig. 11.3).

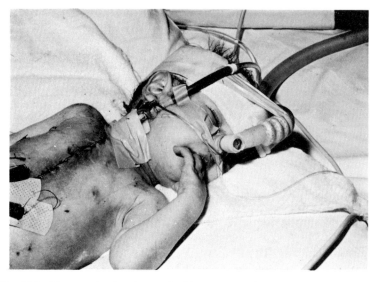

Fig. 11.3 Photograph of a six-month-old baby taken 24 hours after closure of a ventricular septal defect. The patient is breathing spontaneously via a naso-endotracheal tube. There is one intravenous line placed through the internal jugular vein.

When all the vital systems of the patient are stable following return to the intensive care unit, and when the patient is fully awake but sedated, he is transferred from mechanical artificial ventilation to continuous positive airways pressure breathing. This allows the patient to breathe spontaneously; continues to allow accurate monitoring of inspired gas concentrations; and, by including an expiratory resistance in the ventilatory circuit, mitigates against micro-atelectasis, a not uncommon complication following cardiopulmonary bypass. Only when all other vital signs are normal and the patient has shown that he can breathe spontaneously at normal inspiratory pressure with normal inspired gas concentrations is he extubated.

Definitive operations

Of necessity, the descriptions of surgical treatment of congenital malformations must be somewhat abbreviated and they will be given in the appropriate chapters for given malformations. Indications for palliative surgery, when possible or necessary, will be noted, followed by a description of the definitive repair. In order to put the surgical treatment in perspective, an average mortality will be given for each operation; the figure gives a fair indication of current results at the Brompton Hospital and in other major paediatric cardiological referral centres. Finally, this introductory chapter to surgical treatment is concluded with a description of some of the palliative operations which may be necessary.

Palliative operations in the treatment of congenital heart disease
Patients with congenital heart disease can in many instances be adequately palliated by extra-cardiac procedures. Palliation can be performed for patients who have diminished pulmonary blood flow, inadequate communication between pulmonary and systemic circulations, or excessive pulmonary blood flow; the first two cause cyanosis and the third causes pulmonary plethora with congestive cardiac failure.

1. *Decreased pulmonary blood flow.* In patients with obstruction to blood flow to the lungs, a systemic artery/pulmonary artery anastomosis can be constructed to allow an increase in the flow of blood to the pulmonary arteries. This can be carried out by:
   a anastomosing one or other subclavian artery to the right or left pulmonary artery (Blalock–Taussig shunt).
   b anastomosing the right pulmonary artery to the back of the ascending aorta (Waterton shunt).
   c anastomosing the left pulmonary artery to the front of the first part of the descending thoracic aorta (Potts shunt).
   d using an artificial tube prosthesis to connect the aorta or subclavian artery to one or other of the pulmonary arteries.
The systemic artery/pulmonary artery anastomosis of choice is still that of Blalock and Taussig, the first palliative operation performed for patients with reduced pulmonary blood flow. This anastomosis allows an appropriate amount of blood to pass into the pulmonary arteries,

thereby avoiding the complications of excessive flow and pulmonary vascular disease which are sometimes seen in the other forms of anastomosis.

2. *Palliation for lack of intracardiac mixing.* In patients with complete transposition of the great arteries there is inadequate communication between the pulmonary and systemic circulations, to alleviate this surgical atrial septectomy can be performed as a closed procedure in which part of the atrial septum is excised (Blalock–Hanlon septostomy). This operation has a not inconsiderable mortality and is rarely performed except in older life, since patients with transposition of the great arteries requiring palliation are now successfully palliated by means of the balloon atrial septostomy (see Chapter 27).

3. *Excessive pulmonary flow.* In patients with anomalies which result in excessive blood flow to the lungs, reduction of flow can be performed by banding or narrowing the main pulmonary artery. This is carried out by means of a constricting tape that attempts to reduce the distal pulmonary artery pressure to 30 per cent of the proximal pulmonary artery pressure.

12 The asymptomatic child with a heart murmur

The asymptomatic child with a cardiac murmur presents a common clinical problem. Many normal children, most children with minor cardiac defects, and some with major defects come into this category. Not every child with a murmur can be referred to a paediatric cardiologist. Selection of patients for such referral depends on an appraisal of clinical findings, in particular the timing, loudness, and point of maximal intensity of the murmur. Even more important, however, is evaluation of the rest of the cardiovascular system, such as the pulses, cardiac impulse, and heart sounds.

Systolic murmurs

The loud basal systolic murmur

Most loud systolic murmurs maximal at the high right or left sternal border, especially if accompanied by a thrill, are due to right or left ventricular outflow tract obstruction. Aortic and pulmonary stenosis can usually be differentiated by location and radiation of the murmur, pulmonary stenosis being louder at the high left and aortic stenosis at the high right sternal border. Radiation of the murmur to the neck is more marked with aortic stenosis. Most cases of aortic stenosis have an associated early systolic ejection sound (or click). An aortic ejection sound is usually loudest at the apex (not the second right intercostal space where the murmur is loudest) and has roughly the same pitch as the first heart sound. It sounds, in fact, like a split first heart sound. A pulmonary ejection sound has a higher pitch and is maximal at the high left sternal border. If the first sound is inaudible at the base, a pulmonary ejection sound may seem to be the first heart sound, but its high pitch and clicking quality are characteristic. If the two components of the second sound can be heard easily aortic or pulmonary stenosis is unlikely to be severe. A normal chest X-ray and electrocardiogram are reassuring in the case of pulmonary stenosis but are less so with aortic stenosis.

The soft basal systolic murmur

A soft basal systolic murmur is found with mild pulmonary or aortic stenosis, coarctation of the aorta, or an atrial septal defect, but may be functional, originating at an arterial valve. The murmur itself is not as helpful in differential diagnosis as are the associated findings. Coarctation, for instance, can be diagnosed by comparing arm and leg pulses. Mild aortic and pulmonary stenosis can be identified by the usually associated early systolic ejection sound and by the striking increase in intensity of the murmur which occurs with exercise. An atrial septal defect is the most frequently missed important congenital cardiac anomaly, since the basal systolic murmur is soft and the child seems healthy. If an atrial septal defect is present the second sound remains split throughout the respiratory cycle and is split even after forced expiration.

If pulses and cardiac impulse are normal, if there is no early systolic ejection sound, and if the second sound is normally split, a soft basal systolic murmur is usually functional and of no significance.

A loud systolic murmur at the low left sternal border

In an asymptomatic child, a loud systolic murmur maximal at the low left sternal border is almost always due to a ventricular septal defect. There may or may not be an associated thrill. If the left-to-right shunt is large, flow across the mitral valve will be increased and a rumbling mid-diastolic murmur will be present at the apex. Such a murmur should be sought in children suspected of having a ventricular septal defect; its presence suggests a pulmonary flow at least twice systemic. A chest X-ray and electrocardiogram should be obtained in every child with a loud mid or low left sternal border systolic murmur. The intensity of the pulmonary component of the second sound and degree of right ventricular hypertrophy on ECG are more important than the intensity of the murmur in deciding if a child with a suspected ventricular septal defect requires cardiac catheterization.

The soft low left sternal border murmur

A soft low or mid left sternal border systolic murmur may be functional or represent a very small ventricular septal defect. These entities are best differentiated by the characteristic quality of the functional (innocent) murmur which has been called 'vibratory' or 'like a twanging string', neither of which terms describes it particularly well. Like an old friend, the murmur is quite easy to recognize but surprisingly difficult to describe. It tends to be low-pitched and buzzing with an intensity that varies, being louder during febrile illnesses. The murmur of a tiny ventricular septal defect is high pitched and may be pansystolic or may end well before the second sound. Again, normality of the second sound must be confirmed.

Apical systolic murmur

A systolic murmur which is maximal at the apex is nearly always due to mitral regurgitation. In most cases the murmur is pansystolic but it may be late systolic, especially if the mitral regurgitation is due to mitral valve leaflet prolapse. If the mitral regurgitation is severe the apical impulse will be overactive and there will be an apical mid-diastolic rumble. The rumble is due to large flow across the valve in diastole, an inevitable consequence of major systolic regurgitation to the left atrium. The systolic murmur itself tells little about the severity of the regurgitation. If mitral regurgitation is mild the chest X-ray and electrocardiogram will be normal. If severe, cardiomegaly, left atrial enlargement, and upper lobe blood diversion may be present. The electrocardiogram may show left ventricular hypertrophy and often left atrial enlargement.

Diastolic murmurs

An isolated diastolic murmur in an asymptomatic child is rare. The mid-diastolic flow murmur of a large atrial or ventricular septal defect will be accompanied by a more prominent systolic murmur. Children with a diastolic murmur due to mitral stenosis are usually symptomatic. Isolated early diastolic murmurs may be found with mild aortic or pulmonary incompetence. The murmur of aortic regurgitation is high-pitched and decrescendo and is maximal along the mid left sternal border. It is best heard during squatting or with the child sitting with the breath held in expiration but is often faint and can easily be missed. Isolated pulmonary regurgitation is rare. The murmur is typically short and soft and is maximal at the mid left sternal border. It is usually louder with the child in a recumbent position.

Continuous murmurs

A continuous murmur maximal at the base (typically under the left clavicle) in a well child is most probably a venous hum or the murmur of a persistent ductus arteriosus. Either may be loud or soft. A wide pulse pressure will be present if the ductus is large but absent if the ductus is small; hence differentiation has often to be made solely on auscultatory criteria. Much has been made of the differential value of a change in intensity of a venous hum with head turning or pressure over the jugular veins. A much easier and more reliable manoeuvre is simply to have the child lie down. A jugular venous hum disappears; the murmur of a ductus persists.

Other causes of a basal continuous murmur are flow through systemic pulmonary collateral arteries in pulmonary atresia with ventricular septal defect, truncal incompetence, or flow through systemic collaterals in coarctation of the aorta. All illustrate the importance of the rest of the physical examination in regard to assessing the significance of a murmur; thus with the first two conditions there will be a single second sound (with or without cyanosis) and with the latter decreased or absent femoral pulses. Less easy to distinguish from a ductus arteriosus are a small ventricular defect plus aortic incompetence, a small aorto-pulmonary window, or a coronary artery or sinus of Valsalva fistula. All children with a continuous murmur not abolished by lying down (with or without head turning) should be investigated further.

13 Normal embryogenesis of the heart

Before dealing with specific malformations, an account will be given of the embryological development of the normal heart, for without this it is difficult to understand the morphogenesis and anatomy of any but the simplest anomalies.

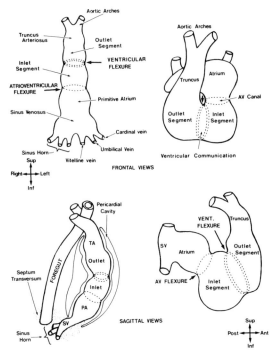

Fig. 13.1 The mechanics of ventricular looping. The upper panels show, on the left, the heart tube prior to looping and on the right the tube after looping. The lower panels show corresponding views seen laterally. Looping occurs between the atrium and the inlet segment of the ventricle and between the inlet and outlet segments of the ventricular loop. The atrioventricular canal is shown as a single dotted circle while the ventricular communication is shown as a double dotted circle.

TA = truncus arteriosus; PA = primitive atrium; SV = sinus venosus; AV = atrioventricular.

The 'compasses' show orientation.

Development will be considered from the stages at which the heart is a straight tube (Fig. 13.1). Originally this single tube was derived from fusion of paired symmetrical primordia. The tube shows several dilatations along its length. The venous dilatation of sinus venosus is embedded in the substance of the septum transversum, in which the liver also develops. Veins enter the sinus venosus on each side from the placenta (umbilical veins), the yolk sac (vitelline veins), and the embryo itself (cardinal veins). The sinus venosus then communicates with a series of dilatations in the tube, namely the primitive atrium, the ventricular component which comprises two dilatations and truncus arteriosus (Fig. 13.1). The distal end of the truncus, the aortic sac, gives rise to a series of aortic arches which encircle the developing pharynx to enter the descending aorta. The whole tube is invaginated in the pericardial

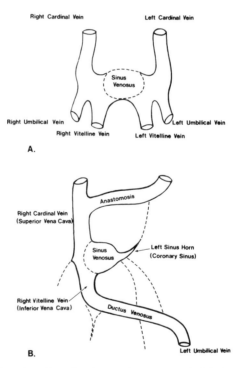

Fig. 13.2   The alterations that take place at the venous end of the heart following the formation of left to right anastomoses. (A) shows the sinus venosus and its tributaries prior to formation of these anastomoses. (B) shows the situation after their formation.

cavity. At this stage, the embryo is approximately six weeks of age and measures approximately 10 mm.

The next stage of development is cardiac looping. The sinus venosus, being firmly embedded in the septum transversum, serves as the fixed end of the tube. Differential growth brings the primitive atrium back towards the sinus venosus and produces a right-angled flexure between the atrium and the inlet component of the ventricular segment. A further flexure of 180° is produced in the ventricular segment itself, so that the truncus comes to lie in front of and to the right of the atrioventricular canal (Fig. 13.1). This looping usually occurs to the right, and is termed dextro-(*d*-) ventricular looping.

After the completion of looping, the heart begins to assume a shape comparable with the formed heart, but is still composed of a single tube. Septation is therefore the next process of development, and occurs within the atrial, ventricular, and truncal segments of the heart.

Changes in the atrial segment are dependent upon reorganization of the venous system. The originally bilaterally symmetrical system becomes lateralized by development of left-to-right anastomoses in the head and abdominal regions (Fig. 13.2). The superior anastomosis is between the cardinal systems, so that the left superior cardinal vein is drained into the right vein and thence to the sinus venosus. The abdominal changes involve both vitelline and umbilical systems. A new channel, the ductus venosus, connects the left umbilical to the right

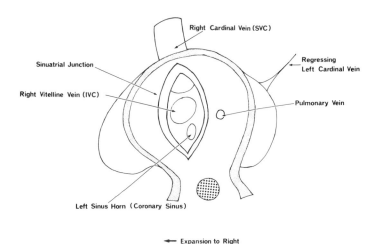

Fig. 13.3 The effect of the development of the left to right anastomoses on the drainage of the sinus venosus to the primitive atrium.

vitelline vein, and the latter persists as the portion of the inferior vena cava which enters the sinus venosus. The other channels regress, parts of the vitelline veins becoming incorporated into the portal system. Following this reorganization, all blood is drained to the right side of

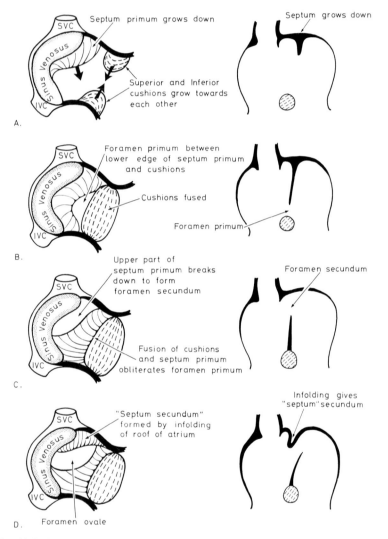

Fig. 13.4   The mode of development of the atrial septum. The left hand diagrams show a lateral view while the right hand diagrams show a frontal section through the atrial chambers.

the sinus venosus through the prospective superior vena cava (right cardinal vein) and inferior vena cava (right vitelline vein). The left side of the sinus regresses, persisting only as the coronary sinus and oblique vein (Fig. 13.2).

With this development of right dominance, there is a shift to the right side of the sinuatrial junction, which then opens entirely to the right side of the primitive atrium (Fig. 13.3). A new venous channel, the primary pulmonary vein, grows from the left side of the primitive atrium. Concomitant with right-sided shift of the sinuatrial junction there is also rightward expansion of the atrioventricular junction. The expanding atrioventricular canal is at the same time septated by the formation of opposing superior and inferior endocardial cushions. The midline fusion of these cushions divides the canal into right and left atrioventricular orifices (Fig. 13.4). The primitive atrium is now septated by formation of a midline septum, the septum primum. This structure originally grows down from the roof of the atrium between the sinuatrial junction and the pulmonary vein. As it grows down, its crescentic lower edge approximates to the fusing endocardial cushions. The gap between this margin and the cushions is the ostium primum (Fig. 13.4B). Fusion between the septum primum and the cushions obliterates the ostium primum. At the same time, the upper margin of the septum breaks down to provide a continuing interatrial communication. This upper communication is the foramen secundum. An infolding of the right side of the primitive atrial wall then forms between the sinuatrial junction and the site of origin of the septum primum. This infolding covers the foramen secundum and overlaps the persisting lower portion of the septum primum. The slit-like gap between the two is the foramen ovale (Fig. 13.4D). Tissues of the sinuatrial junction usually persist as thin valve-like structures. These are the sinus valves and they function during fetal life to direct the richly oxygenated inferior caval blood from the placenta through the foramen ovale to the left atrium.

During this period, growth of the primary pulmonary vein has also been taking place. This single channel grows out towards the developing lung buds, themselves outgrowths from the foregut (Fig. 13.5). A separate plexus of pulmonary veins develops within the lung beds from the splanchnic venous plexus which originally surrounded the foregut. If development is normal, the single primary pulmonary vein joins up with these secondary intrapulmonary plexuses (Fig. 13.5(2)). The single channel together with some of the pulmonary veins is then reabsorbed into the substance of the newly formed left atrium. This

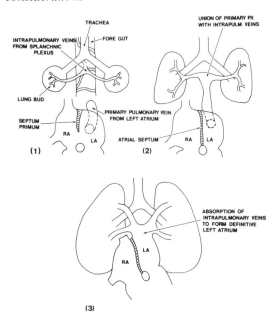

Fig. 13.5   The mode of development of connexions between the intrapulmonary veins developing within the lung bud and the primary pulmonary vein developing from the left atrium.

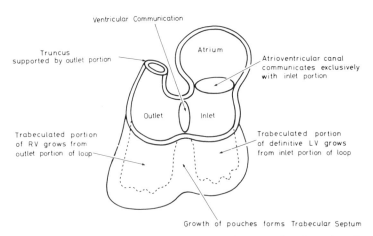

Fig. 13.6   The development of the trabecular ventricular portions from the primary heart tube.

reabsorption takes place up to the second division of the pulmonary veins, so that eventually four discrete channels open into the definitive left atrium (Fig. 13.5(3)).

Following looping, pouches are formed from both the inlet and outlet portions of the primary heart tube (Fig. 13.6). The pouch formed from the inlet segment will eventually form the trabecular zone of the left ventricle while the pouch formed from the outlet portion will form the trabecular zone of the right ventricle. Excavation of these pouches produces the trabecular septum which forms the lower rim of the communication between inlet and outlet parts of the ventricular loop (Fig. 13.6). The upper rim is the inner heart curvature. At this stage, the entire input from the atrioventricular canals drains to the left ventricular trabecular zone while the truncus, and hence both outlets, is supported above the right ventricular trabecular zone. Concomitant with septation of the atrioventricular canal by the endocardial cushions there is expansion and shift of the inlet segment so that its right side becomes committed to the trabecular zone of right ventricular type. At the same time an inlet septum is formed between the right and left atrioventricular orifices so that the right ventricle then has an inlet and both outlets while the left ventricle has only an inlet (Fig. 13.7). Blood entering the left ventricle must reach the developing aortic outflow

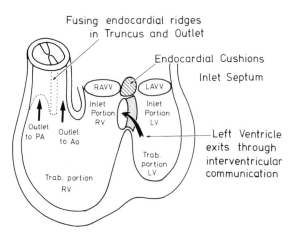

Fig. 13.7 The appearance of the primary heart tube and its trabecular pouches following transfer of the inlet portion of the right ventricle (RAVV right atrioventricular valve, LAVV left atrioventricular valve).

tract by passing through the foramen bounded by the inlet septum, the trabecular septum and the inner heart curvature (Fig. 13.8, upper diagram). Development of the ventricles is then completed by transfer of the developing aortic outflow tract to the left ventricle, producing the situation where each ventricle has an inlet, trabecular, and outlet portion (Fig. 13.8, lower diagram). In this same period of growth the outlet part of the ventricular loop and the truncus have been septated by fusion of opposing endocardial ridges. Transfer of the aorta to the left ventricle results in the outlet septum being brought into line with the trabecular and inlet septa, but following transfer a communication still persists between the aortic outflow tract and the right ventricle. This is the interventricular communication which is closed by growth of tissue from the endocardial cushions (Fig. 13.8). During the same period the inner heart curvature has become effaced to permit the developing aortic outflow tract to fall back into the left ventricle. Initially, therefore, both developing arterial valves at the outlet-truncal junction are supported by the outlet segment of the ventricular loop. During transfer of the aorta the posterior part of this segment,

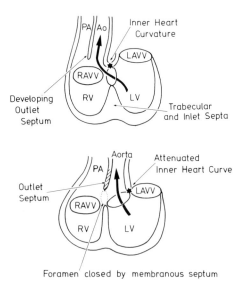

Fig. 13.8 The mode of transfer of the aorta to the left ventricle consequent upon absorption and attenuation of the inner heart curve. Note the position of the star on the inner heart curvature and the fact that the communication between left ventricle and aorta never closes. The foramen which is closed by the membranous septum is a new 'hole'.

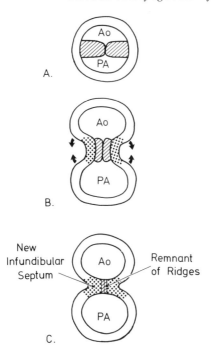

Fig. 13.9 The formation of the definitive septum between aorta and pulmonary outflow tract by coalescence of the opposing walls of the vessels rather than from the endocardial ridges themselves (cross-hatched area).

the inner heart curve, is attenuated so that the developing aortic valve is brought into continuity with the developing mitral valve.

The endocardial ridges which separate the outlet portion of the ventricular loop continue into the truncus. Initially disposed in spiral fashion, these ridges straighten out as they fuse to separate the aorta and pulmonary artery. The definitive septum which separates the outflow tracts is not derived from the initial endocardial ridges, but is formed by coalescence of the walls of the outflow tracts (Fig. 13.9). It is the infundibular septum. Where the inner heart curvature persists as a muscular structure, it is the ventriculo-infundibular fold (Fig. 13.10). The tissue which eventually closes the interventricular communication becomes the membranous part of the ventricular septum. The definitive ventricular septum is therefore derived from four sources, namely, the trabecular septum, inlet septum, infundibular septum, and membranous septum (Fig. 13.10).

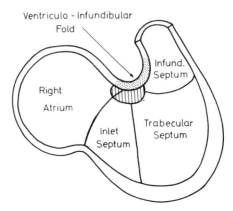

Fig. 13.10 The definitive parts of the ventricular septum. The muscular septum has three components and is completed by the fibrous membranous septum (cross-hatched area).

Septation of the ventricular outflow tracts by the outlet septum and truncal septum has been described. The ridges which fuse to form the conus septum also septate the truncus. Although originally arranged in a spiral fashion, when fused they form a straight septum. The aortic sac is septated by the down-growing aortic-pulmonary septum. This fuses with the truncal septum in such a way that the aortic outflow tract is connected to the fourth aortic arch, while the pulmonary outflow tract becomes attached to the sixth arch. Following fusion, the tension generated by the original spiral disposition of the ridges within the outlet and truncus is transmitted to the aortic arches so that the great arteries spiral around each other as they ascend from the heart. During fetal life the sixth arch connects to the descending aorta as the ductus arteriosus.

The atrioventricular valves are formed by delamination of the superficial layers of the ventricular inlet portions. The arterial valves are formed at the original outlet-truncal junction. Initially both atrioventricular valves are separated from both arterial valves by the ventriculo-infundibular fold (inner heart curvature). Following transfer of the aorta to the left ventricle, the fold is no longer present between the aortic and mitral valves, hence the normal finding of aortic-mitral continuity. In contrast, the fold persists between the tricuspid and pulmonary valves in the right ventricle and is reinforced by the infundibular septum. These two structures form the normal crista supraventricularis and result in tricuspid-pulmonary discontinuity.

References

Anderson, K. R. and Anderson, R. H. (1978). Growth and development of the cardiovascular system. (A) Anatomical development. In *Scientific foundations of paediatrics* (ed. J. A. Davis and J. Dobbing) 2nd edn. Heinemann, London. In the press.

Anderson, R. H. (1978). Another look at cardiac embryology. In *Progress in cardiology* 7 (ed. P. N. Yu and J. F. Goodwin), pp. 1–54. Lea & Febiger, New York.

Goor, D. A. and Lillehei, C. W. (1975). *Congenital malformations of the heart*, pp. 38–88, Grune and Stratton, New York.

Van Mierop, L. H. S. (1969). *Embryology in the Ciba Collection of Medical Illustrations. Volume 5: The Heart* (ed. F. H. Netter), pp. 112–126. Ciba, New York.

Part II
Specific conditions and their management

14 Atrial septal defect (ASD)

Chapters 14 to 45 should be read in conjunction with the general chapters on physical examination, modes of presentation, and differential diagnosis etc. We have not thought it productive in these chapters to detail all physical findings for each anomaly but only those of principal diagnostic importance.

Anatomy and embryology
Defects in the atrial septum can be divided into ostium primum defects, patent foramen ovale, defects in the floor of the fossa ovalis (secundum defects), and sinus venosus defects (Fig. 14.1).

The ostium primum defect is a consequence of incomplete fusion

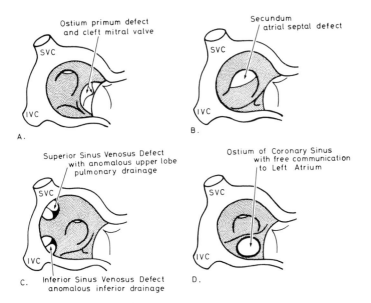

Fig. 14.1 The type of atrial septal defect. (A) shows an ostium primum defect, (B) shows a secundum defect and (C) shows the sinus venosus type of defect. (D) shows the drainage of a coronary sinus to the right atrium with free communication to the left atrium. It is questionable if this should be considered as an atrial septal defect.

between the down-growing septum primum and the endocardial cushions. It has all the stigmata of an atrioventricular canal malformation (see Chapter 20). Lack of fusion of the endocardial cushions themselves is usually present also, resulting in a cleft of the mitral valve (Fig. 14.1A). The patent foramen ovale and ostium secundum defects are both in the site of the fetal inter-atrial communication. The former is present when the flap valve of the fossa ovalis and its limbus can be apposed to close the defect, thus preventing any left-to-right shunt. When this is not possible, a defect is always present, usually termed a secundum defect (Fig. 14.1B). The sinus venosus defect can be considered as a consequence of anomalous insertion of the right pulmonary veins, so that in addition to a defect in the atrial septum at least the right upper pulmonary vein enters the superior vena cava, or else the right lower pulmonary vein enters the inferior vena cava (Fig. 14.1C). A further condition often referred to as an atrial septal defect is an unroofed coronary sinus (Fig. 14.1D), but in this anomaly the apparent atrial septal defect is the true ostium of the coronary sinus.

Incidence

A probe patent foramen ovale is a chance autopsy finding in 25 per cent of subjects. It is of no clinical significance and will not be discussed further. Of the atrial defects, the commonest is the ostium secundum defect, which forms the commonest congenital cardiac defect found in adults. After the first year of life, it is seen in approximately 10 per cent of children with congenital heart disease presenting for the first time to a referral centre.

Clinical findings

Presentation

The majority of patients with an isolated secundum defect are asymptomatic and the anomaly is discovered during routine examination. If the defect, and hence the left-to-right shunt, is particularly large, minimal dyspnoea on exertion may be present. Under 2 per cent present with heart failure in the neonatal period, and a small proportion present in adult life with breathlessness and an irregular pulse due to the onset of atrial fibrillation. Effort dyspnoea is more likely when mitral incompetence complicates a primum defect.

Cyanosis is uncommon but may occur due to shunt reversal from pulmonary vascular disease (Eisenmenger syndrome). In younger patients, streaming of the inferior vena caval return through a secundum (or inferior sinus venosus) defect occurs rarely and will also result in cyanosis.

Abnormal findings in all large atrial septal defects include a prominent parasternal impulse due to hypertrophy and dilatation of the right ventricle, possible pulmonary artery pulsation in the second or third left intercostal space, but a normal apical impulse (unless there is associated severe mitral incompetence in a primum defect).

Physical examination
The most specific physical finding resulting from an atrial septal defect, is found at auscultation and consists of wide fixed splitting of the second heart sound. The left-to-right shunt at atrial level causes distension of the right ventricle which has to eject a greater stroke volume. This delays pulmonary valve closure. On inspiration, not only pulmonary but also aortic valve closure are further delayed as the venous return to both ventricles is increased. An ejection systolic murmur maximal in the second left intercostal space is caused by increased flow across the pulmonary valve. A mid-diastolic tricuspid flow murmur may be heard at the lower sternal edge when the pulmonary systemic flow ratio is greater than 2·5:1. An additional auscultatory finding may be an ejection click (pulmonary). In ostium primum defects the apical pansystolic murmur of mitral incompetence is frequently heard owing to the cleft mitral valve.

On *chest X-ray* the degree of cardiomegaly depends on the magnitude of the shunt. The ventricular shadow and main pulmonary artery may be dilated more so with increasing age, but the left atrium will not be enlarged unless there is additional mitral incompetence. In young patients plethora may be absent despite large shunts, although later the vessels become more prominent. In the presence of severe pulmonary vascular disease, gross dilatation of the proximal pulmonary artery is apparent (Fig. 14.2). The ECG exhibits sinus rhythm except in older patients who have developed atrial fibrillation. P-waves are usually normal. The finding of a prolonged P–R interval (first-degree block) is usually indicative of an ostium primum defect. Similarly, a superior QRS axis strongly suggests a primum defect though both these features have been observed in secundum defects. Typically in the latter, the QRS axis is to the right of $+90°$ (right axis deviation). An incomplete right bundle branch block pattern, rSR in V_4R and V_1, is a feature of all atrial septal defects, but can be found in normal subjects. Absence of this pattern when the rest of the clinical assessment indicates an atrial septal defect should raise the suspicion of

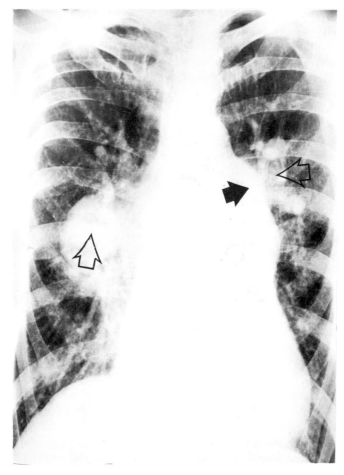

Fig. 14.2 Chest radiograph from a 43-year-old patient with an atrial septal defect and severe pulmonary vascular disease. There is gross dilatation of the main (solid arrow) and proximal (open arrows) pulmonary arteries with peripheral pruning.

hemianomalous pulmonary venous drainage. Definite right ventricular hypertrophy tends to follow an increased pulmonary vascular resistance.

Cardiac catheterization will reveal a step-up in oxygen saturation at atrial level usually with minimal elevation of right ventricular and pulmonary artery pressures. A step-up in oxygen saturation between high and low superior vena caval samples suggests a sinus venosus

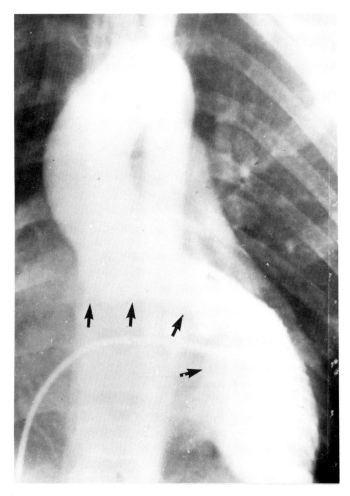

Fig. 14.3 Left ventricular angiogram (frontal projection) in a patient with an ostium primum atrial septal defect. The arrows outline the 'goose-neck' deformity demonstrable during diastole. This appearance is produced by undyed blood coming through the abnormally positioned mitral valve. The latter results from shortening of the inflow portion of the ventricular septum, while the neck of the goose is accentuated by anterior rightward displacement of the aorta (see Fig. 20.2).

defect. When pulmonary vascular disease supervenes, the right-sided pressures increase and eventually right-to-left shunting occurs. An angiogram in the left ventricle will have normal appearances in most secundum defects. In primum defects a 'goose-neck' deformity is present (Fig. 14.3) due to the abnormal position of the mitral valve. Regurgitation of contrast to the atria may occur through the mitral valve cleft. The atrial septum can be profiled by using the 'four-chamber view', namely 45° left anterior oblique and 45° cranio-caudal tilt. Contrast injected into left atrium or optimally right upper pulmonary vein then allows the size and position of the defect to be demonstrated.

Treatment

Unless the shunt is minimal ($Q_p:Q_s < 1.5:1$), all secundum or sinus venosus defects should be closed surgically by direct suture or by means of a Dacron or pericardial patch. It is uncommon for this to be required in infancy. Treatment of the sinus venosus defect is by the placement of an interatrial baffle which redirects blood from the right pulmonary veins into the left atrium. The hospital mortality for these conditions is 0–2 per cent.

Primum defects pose considerably more problems. The intimate relationship between the atrioventricular conduction tissue and the defect makes traumatic heart block an important surgical complication. In general, surgery is undertaken when there are symptoms or if the shunt is large and there is a greater risk of developing pulmonary vascular disease. Palliation of this defect is inappropriate, and one-stage corrective surgery is performed, regardless of size or age. Surgical correction consists of repair of the cleft of the anterior leaflet in the mitral valve, and closure of the atrial septum with a dacron or pericardial patch. Since the most inferior part of the atrial septal defect is the atrioventricular annulus, it is necessary to attach the base of the patch to the base of the septal leaflet of the mitral valve, avoiding the adjacent area of the atrioventricular node. When closing the cleft in the mitral valve leaflet, it may become apparent that complete closure of the cleft will cause shortening of the leaflet tissue, with ensuing mitral incompetence. In such instances a compromise must be reached, allowing only partial closure of the cleft, since a moderate amount of mitral valve incompetence is preferable to mitral valve replacement in these patients, who are frequently young. The hospital mortality of this condition is 0–5 per cent.

References

Bedford, D. E., Papp, C., and Parkinson, J. (1941). Atrial septal defect. *British Heart Journal* **27**, 90.

DuShane, J. W., Weidman, W. H., Brandenburg, R. O., and Kirklin, J. W. (1960). Differentiation of interatrial communications by clinical methods: ostium secundum, ostium primum, common atrium and total anomalous pulmonary venous connection. *Circulation* **21**, 363.

Hunt, C. E. and Lucas, R. V. Jr. (1973). Symptomatic atrial septal defect in infancy. *Circulation* **47**, 1042.

Kaplan, S. (1968). Atrial septal defect. In *Paediatric cardiology* (ed. H. Watson), pp. 376–414. Lloyd Luke, London.

15 Total anomalous pulmonary venous drainage

Anatomy and embryology

During normal development, the common pulmonary vein grows from the left side of the primitive atrium to make contact with the confluence of the intrapulmonary veins formed *in situ*. Should this union not occur, the confluence has the capacity to unite with other venous structures. The site of the anomalous junction forms the basis of classification (Fig. 15.1). The major division is into supradiaphragmatic and infradiaphragmatic forms. In supradiaphragmatic drainage, the

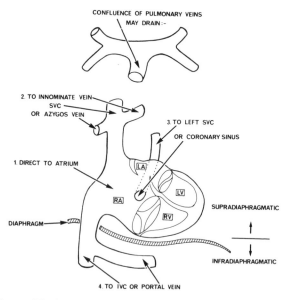

Fig. 15.1 The possible sites of drainage of anomalous pulmonary venous connexion. They are divisible into supra-diaphragmatic and infra-diaphragmatic types with various sites to which the confluence of pulmonary veins may drain.

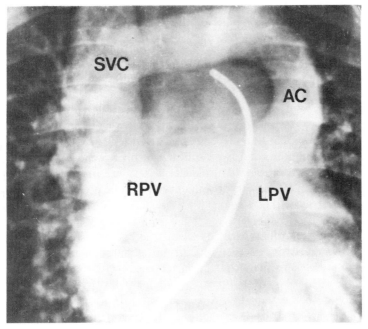

Fig. 15.2 Follow-through from a pulmonary artery injection showing anomalous connexion of the pulmonary venous return. The right and left pulmonary veins (RPV, LPV) drain to an ascending channel (AC) which in turn drains to the superior vena cava (SVC).

confluence forms a common channel which may drain to the superior vena cava (Fig. 15.2), the right atrium directly, the coronary sinus or left superior vena cava, azygos, or innominate veins. Infradiaphragmatic drainage may be direct to the inferior vena cava but is more usually to the portal vein (Fig. 15.1). In isolated total anomalous pulmonary venous drainage an atrial septal defect (or patent foramen ovale) has to be present for blood to reach the left side of the heart. In the infradiaphragmatic group when the ductus venosus (between portal vein and inferior vena cava) closes post-natally, usually by the second or third day, all the pulmonary venous return has to pass through the liver before reaching the right side of the heart. The supradiaphragmatic group may also have obstructed pulmonary venous drainage although not normally as severe as in the infradiaphragmatic group. A likely site is when the ascending common trunk (AC, Fig. 15.2) may be compressed between the left main bronchus and the left pulmonary artery.

Incidence
It is an uncommon condition.

Clinical findings
This anomaly falls into the group of common mixing situations with cyanosis and plethora on chest X-ray (Chapter 9). The mode of presentation is dependent upon the presence or absence of obstruction to pulmonary venous return. In the absence of obstruction, clinical features are similar to those of a large atrial septal defect (prominent parasternal impulse and fixed splitting of the second sound), but in most children cyanosis and in all arterial desaturation (confirmed by a $Po_2 < 150$ mmHg in 100 per cent oxygen) will be present. Pulmonary and even tricuspid flow murmurs are heard when pulmonary venous drainage is totally unobstructed, but if the pulmonary artery pressure is elevated the murmurs disappear while the pulmonary component of the second sound becomes louder. Infradiaphragmatic drainage is almost always obstructed and presents in the first two weeks of life with cyanosis and dyspnoea. On auscultation in this group a very loud pulmonary component to the second sound will be heard.

The chest X-ray in obstructed infradiaphragmatic total anomalous pulmonary venous drainage will show pulmonary oedema characteristically with normal heart size; it may be difficult to distinguish this condition from hyaline membrane disease or neonatal pneumonitis. Here again arterial blood gas analysis during administration of 100 per cent oxygen is invaluable in differential diagnosis. When anomalous drainage is to the superior vena cava the abnormal vein gives rise to the so-called snowman or cottage loaf appearance (broad upper mediastinum), neither of which the X-ray closely resembles! Despite plethora heart size may be normal.

The *ECG* shows an axis to the right of normal and right ventricular hypertrophy, very marked in the presence of obstruction. Cardiac catheterization reveals a step-up in oxygen saturation at right atrial or superior vena caval level. Left atrial samples are desaturated and a common mixing situation is indicated by the finding of similar saturations in both ventricles, aorta, and pulmonary artery. The pulmonary arterial and right ventricular systolic pressures are elevated, greater elevation being present with obstruction to pulmonary venous return. The precise site of anomalous drainage is determined by angiography, either by retrograde catheterization of the anomalous channel from the right atrium (Fig. 15.3) or more commonly by injection into the pulmonary artery and follow-through (Fig. 15.2). Infradiaphragmatic

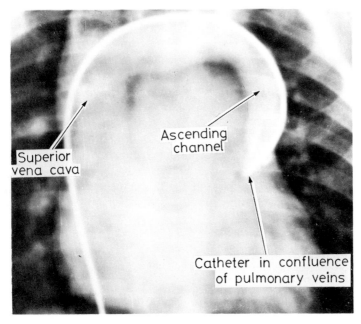

Fig. 15.3   Angiogram obtained via the right atrium by injecting into the confluence of an anomalously connecting pulmonary venous circuit.

drainage to the portal vein can be demonstrated by injection of contrast medium through a catheter introduced into the umbilical vein.

Treatment
Treatment is surgical. The repair varies depending on the type of anomalous connexion.

When the pulmonary veins drain to the coronary sinus the latter is opened by cutting back its superior wall into the atrial septal defect and thereby diverting all blood from the pulmonary veins into the left atrium. A baffle is then placed to incorporate the coronary sinus into the atrial septal defect.

In the supracardiac type of anomalous drainage the horizontal collecting vein is placed retropericardially, and is immediately posterior to the posterior surface of the wall of the left atrium. The horizontal collecting vein usually drains into the left superior vena cava, which in turn drains directly to the innominate vein and thence to the right superior vena cava. Correction of this defect is performed by making an incision in the anterior surface of the horizontal collecting vein, and the posterior surface of the wall of the left atrium. An anastomosis is then constructed connecting the left atrium to the horizontal collecting vein. When this is complete, the left superior vena cava is ligated.

In the infracardiac type of drainage the common collecting vein is in the vertical plane. A similar anastomosis as constructed for supracardiac drainage is performed between the front of the vertical vein and the back of the left atrium, but in this instance the incision is somewhat oblique.

Successful outcome in all these anomalies also depends upon adequate left atrial size. If the left atrium is small, pulmonary venous obstruction may persist.

The mortality is 15 per cent to 25 per cent for nonobstructed anomalous drainage but up to 50 per cent for obstructed infradiaphragmatic drainage.

References

Burchell, H. B. (1956). Total anomalous pulmonary venous drainage: Clinical and physiologic patterns. *Mayo Clinic Proceedings* **31**, 161.

DeLisle, G., Ando, M., Calder, A. L., Zuberbuhler, J. R., Rochenmacher, S., Alday, L. E., Mangino, O., Van Praagh, S., and Van Praagh, R. (1976). Total anomalous pulmonary venous connection: Report of 93 autopsied cases with emphasis on diagnostic and surgical considerations. *American Heart Journal* **91**, 99.

Edwards, J. E. (1953). Pathologic and developmental considerations in anomalous pulmonary venous connection. *Mayo Clinic Proceedings* **28**, 441.

Neill, C. A. (1956). Development of the pulmonary veins with reference to the embryology of the anomalies of pulmonary venous return. *Paediatrics* **18**, 880.

16 Ebstein's anomaly

Anatomy and embryology

Ebstein's anomaly constitutes a spectrum of abnormalities of the tricuspid valve whereby the effective orifice of the valve is displaced to the junction of inlet and trabecular zones of the right ventricle. Usually there is failure of delamination of the septal and inferior leaflets, which

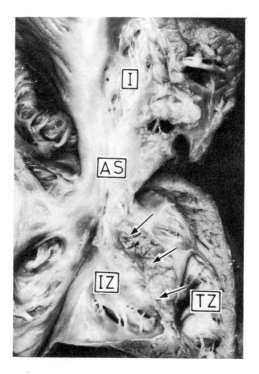

Fig. 16.1 The opened right atrioventricular orifice from a patient with Ebstein's malformation. It shows that the attachment of the septal leaflet of the tricuspid valve is displaced to the junction of the inlet (IZ) and trabecular (TZ) zones of the right ventricle (arrows). The valve tissue is heaped up at this point. Note that the antero-superior leaflet (AS) and inferior leaflet (I) of the valve are dysplastic, the inferior leaflet also being attached to the parietal wall of the ventricle.

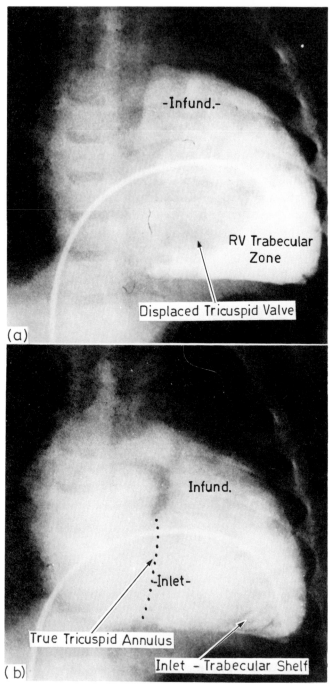

Fig. 16.2 Right ventricular angiograms from a patient with Ebstein's malformation. (a) is taken during ventricular systole when the contrast outlines the displaced attachment of the tricuspid leaflet; (b), taken in diastole, shows the true site of the right atrioventricular annulus. Note also the shelf between inlet and trabecular portions of the ventricle.

are adherent to the wall of the inlet portion. The inlet portion therefore becomes part of the right atrium and is often thin walled and dilated. The antero-superior leaflet is normally attached to the annulus but is abnormally attached inferiorly to the inlet–trabecular junction, which is frequently heaped up to form a prominent shelf (Fig. 16.1). Because of the abnormal attachment the valve is stenotic and may also be regurgitant. The infundibulum may be normal, dilated, or hyper-trophied. An atrial septal defect or patent foramen ovale is commonly present.

Incidence
The anomaly is rare.

Clinical findings
Clinical manifestations vary with the severity of malattachment of the valve. About half the affected individuals present in the neonatal period with cyanosis. They have a quiet heart and few, if any, abnormal findings on auscultation. The chest X-ray shows cardiomegaly, often extreme, and pulmonary oligaemia. *ECG* may show abnormalities of conduction varying from a prolonged P–R interval with right bundle branch block to the Wolff–Parkinson–White syndrome. At *cardiac catheterization* a right-to-left shunt at atrial level is detected in the presence of normal or low pressures in the right ventricle and pulmo-nary artery. Angiocardiography demonstrates the displacement of the tricuspid valve attachment to the junction of the inlet and trabecular components of the right ventricle (Fig. 16.1). Right atrial and right ventricular angiography (Fig. 16.2) confirm the diagnosis, although even at this stage distinction from Uhl's anomaly (parchment right ventricle) and a congenitally dysplastic but normally attached tricuspid valve may be difficult.

Many older patients with a minor '*forme fruste*' of Ebstein's anomaly are asymptomatic or present with paroxysmal supraventricular tachycardia usually related to accessory conduction pathways (see Chapter 45) or atrial fibrillation. Depending on the magnitude of the atrial right-to-left shunt, others present with increasing cyanosis, effort tolerance or even right-sided failure. On examination the cardiac impulse is diffuse and pulses may be of diminished volume. Prominent A or V waves may be seen in distended neck veins. Auscultation reveals a widely split first sound due to delayed tricuspid valve closure, as well as a high-pitched late opening snap from delayed tricuspid valve opening. Scratchy diastolic murmurs and the pansystolic murmur of tricuspid incompetence may also be heard. Cardiomegaly affecting particularly the right atrium, and pulmonary oligaemia are again seen on *chest X-ray*. On *ECG* atrioventricular conduction disturbances, right bundle branch block, and giant P-waves may be seen. At *cardiac catheterization* right atrial pressure is elevated and right ventricular pressure normal or low, although large presystolic waves from the right atrium may be transmitted to the right ventricle or even pulmonary artery. Using an intracardiac electrode, right ventricular electrical activity may be detected in a region where there is a right atrial pressure pulse, thus demonstrating atrialization of part of the right ventricle.

Treatment

Palliation of this condition cannot easily be performed, except for closure of an associated atrial septal defect. The primary aim in surgical correction is to obtain a competent tricuspid valve, allowing forward flow of blood from the right ventricle to the pulmonary artery without damaging the conducting tissue. This can be achieved either by annuloplastic repair of the tricuspid valve, with excision of redundant atrialized ventricular tissue, or else by insertion of a prosthetic valve. The results of surgery are not satisfactory at present. A major complication of surgery is damage to the atrioventricular conduction tissue. The hospital mortality for the condition is 20–30 per cent.

References

Bahnson, H. T., Bauersfield, S. R., and Smith, J. W. (1965). Pathological anatomy and surgical correction of Ebstein's anomaly. *Circulation* **31 & 32 (Suppl. I)**, 3.

Genton, E. and Blount, G. (1967). The spectrum of Ebstein's anomaly. *American Heart Journal* **73**, 395.

Schiebler, G. L., Gravenstein, G. S., and Van Mierop, L. H. S. (1968). Ebstein's anomaly of the tricuspid valve: Translation of original description with comments. *American Journal of Cardiology* **22**, 867.

Van Mierop, L. H. S., Schiebler, G. L., and Victoria, B. E. (1978). Anomalies of the tricuspid valve resulting in stenosis or incompetence. In *Heart disease in infants, children and adolescents* (ed. A. J. Moss, F. H. Adams, and G. C. Emmanouilides), pp. 262–76. Williams & Wilkins, Baltimore.

17 Hypoplastic right ventricle without pulmonary atresia

Anatomy
The right ventricle is shaped like a cylinder with a smaller than normal tricuspid valve ring. The heavily trabeculated apical portion of the normal right ventricle is severely hypoplastic, but the infundibulum is formed and the communication with the pulmonary trunk is patent. The pulmonary valve is usually normal.

Incidence
The anomaly is rare.

Clinical findings
Cyanosis is the presenting feature, usually in the first year of life. The right ventricle impedes anterograde flow possibly as the tricuspid valve ring is mildly stenotic. Elevation of right atrial pressure leads to right-to-left shunting at atrial level across the foramen ovale or atrial septal defect.

On physical examination, apart from cyanosis there are no striking features, the second heart sound frequently being normal. The *ECG* shows a paucity of right ventricular forces for age. Pulmonary vascular markings on *chest X-ray* will be reduced. The heart size may be markedly increased as a result of right atrial enlargement.

At *cardiac catheterization* left-sided pressures and those in the right ventricle and pulmonary artery will be normal, while that in the right atrium may be elevated. There is right-to-left shunting at atrial level. Angiography is necessary to confirm the diagnosis as the haemodynamic findings of a right-to-left shunt at atrial level with normal right-sided haemodynamics is also found with Uhl's anomaly, congenital tricuspid incompetence, and some Ebstein's anomalies.

Treatment
Treatment can be difficult, although simple closure of the foramen ovale or atrial septal defect is sometimes dramatically successful.

Reference

Haworth, S. G., Shinebourne, E. A., and Miller, G. A. H. (1975). Right to left interatrial shunting with normal right ventricular pressure. A puzzling haemodynamic picture associated with some rare congenital malformations of the right ventricle and tricuspid valve. *British Heart Journal* **37**, 386.

18 Uhl's anomaly

Anatomy
Uhl's anomaly or parchment right ventricle is characterized by almost complete absence of working myocardium in the right ventricle, especially the body of the ventricle. Functional tricuspid incompetence is associated.

Incidence
The anomaly is rare.

Clinical findings
Presentation is similar to that of Ebstein's anomaly with atrialization of the right ventricle, tricuspid incompetence, and a right-to-left shunt at atrial level. Again, gross cardiomegaly with oligaemic lung fields are seen and there is a paucity of right ventricular forces on *ECG*. Differential diagnosis is from Ebstein's anomaly, hypoplastic right ventricle, and tricuspid incompetence. Haemodynamic findings at cardiac catheterization are similar to those of hypoplastic right ventricle and the diagnosis is proven by angiography (Fig. 18.1).

Treatment
Oxygen administration is used to encourage pulmonary vascular resistance to fall postnatally, but no corrective treatment is available.

Reference
Uhl, H. S. M. (1952). A previously undescribed congenital malformation of the heart: almost total absence of the myocardium of the right ventricle. *Bulletin of Johns Hopkins Hospital* **91**, 197.

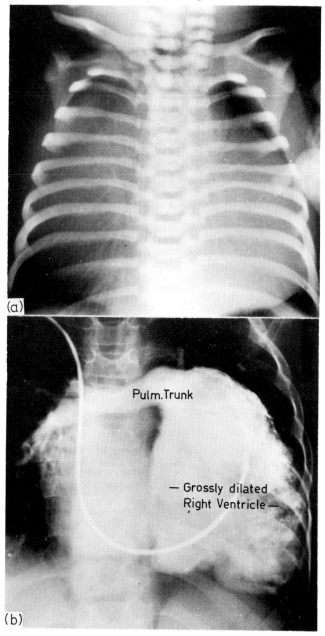

Fig. 18.1 A typical chest X-ray (a) and right ventricular angiogram (b) from a patient with Uhl's anomaly.

19 Cor triatriatum

Anatomy and embryology
The defect is due to failure of re-incorporation of the common pulmonary vein back into the left atrium. The pulmonary veins enter a chamber behind the true left atrium and thence pass through a small or pinhole orifice to the mitral valve and left ventricle (Fig. 19.1).

Incidence
This condition is extremely rare.

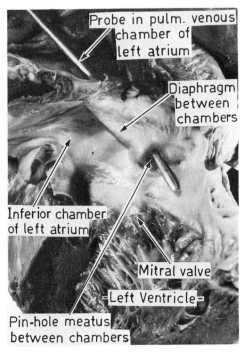

Fig. 19.1 The morphology of the left atrium in a patient with cor triatriatum. Note the membrane formed between the part of the atrium receiving the pulmonary veins and the part above the mitral valve. The only communication between the two is a small pinhole orifice.

Clinical findings

Patients present with breathlessness due to heart failure sometimes with a diastolic murmur reminiscent of mitral stenosis. Breathlessness may be striking when pulmonary venous pressure is high. Signs of pulmonary hypertension will be present. The *ECG* typically shows right ventricular hypertrophy and the *chest X-ray* marked upper lobe blood diversion due to pulmonary venous obstruction. *Echocardiography* can readily distinguish cor triatriatum from other forms of left ventricular inflow obstruction, especially from congenital mitral stenosis, as the mitral valve echogram will be normal. Furthermore the 'membrane' of cor triatriatum may be demonstrated. At *cardiac catheterization* there is a high pulmonary capillary wedge pressure and a low left atrial pressure (entered via a patent foramen ovale). Left atrial blood sampled from here is desaturated.

A high wedge pressure will also be found in congenital mitral stenosis and stenosing ring of the left atrium, but in these conditions, if the left atrium can be entered, the pressure is found to be high. As stated previously, however, these rare anomalies are best differentiated using echocardiography.

Treatment

At surgery, provided that the correct diagnosis has been made, the membrane can easily be incised. The approach is usually via a right atrial incision.

Reference

Van Praagh, R. and Corsini, I. (1969). Cor triatriatum. Pathologic anatomy and a consideration of morphogenesis based on 13 postmortem cases and a study of the pulmonary vein and atrial septum in 83 human embryos. *American Heart Journal* **78**, 379.

20 Common atrioventricular canal

Anatomy and embryology

This defect, the complete form of atrioventricular canal malformation, results from complete failure of normal fusion of the atrioventricular endocardial cushions. It is therefore characterized by presence of a common atrioventricular orifice and valve, an inlet ventricular septal defect, and almost always an ostium primum atrial septal defect (Fig. 20.1). All four cardiac chambers are in communication through these defects. The anomaly is frequently termed a complete endocardial cushion defect. There is characteristic disproportion between the inlet and outlet dimensions of the left ventricle and the aortic valve is malorientated relative to the atrioventricular valve (Fig. 20.2). Further sub-division of the anomaly depends on the anatomy of the bridging anterior valve leaflet and its papillary muscle attachment within the right ventricle. The ostium primum defect in isolation is termed a partial atrioventricular canal malformation (when discrete tricuspid and mitral orifices exist, but the heart has the same basic anatomical structure (see Chapter 14)).

Incidence

This condition is relatively common in patients with trisomy 21 (Down's syndrome or mongolism). Otherwise the anomaly is rare.

Clinical findings

The presentation and physical findings are similar to those of patients with a large ventricular septal defect, with possibly an additional apical pansystolic murmur of 'mitral' regurgitation. As there can be an obligatory shunt from left ventricle through the common valve to the right atrium, as well as 'mitral' regurgitation, infants may present in heart failure in the first or second week of life. The *chest X-ray* shows considerable cardiomegaly, plethora, and a left aortic arch. *ECG* shows sinus rhythm and evidence of atrial and biventricular hypertrophy. First-degree heart block (increased P–R interval) is relatively common. A superior mean frontal QRS axis usually between $0°$ and $-120°$ is the rule and alerts the clinician to the possibility of this diagnosis in all patients with left-to-right shunts (Fig. 8.2). The diag-

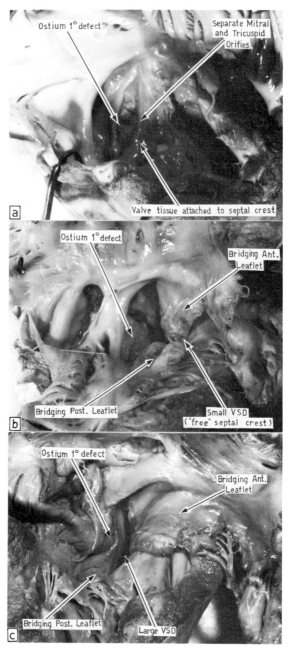

Fig. 20.1 The characteristic morphology of various types of atrioventricular canal malformations. (a) shows an ostium primum defect. The annulus of the mitral and tricuspid orifices is displaced on the septum well into the ventricular cavity with valve tissue attached to the septal crest. The difference between the ostium primum defect and the complete defect is illustrated in (b) and (c) since in these anomalies the valve tissue does not meet on the septal crest due to the presence of bridging anterior and posterior leaflets. There is therefore a ventricular septal defect across the bare area of the ventricular septum. Further sub-division depends upon the attachment of the bridging leaflet, (b) illustrating the so-called Rastelli type A malformation and (c) illustrating the Rastelli type C malformation.

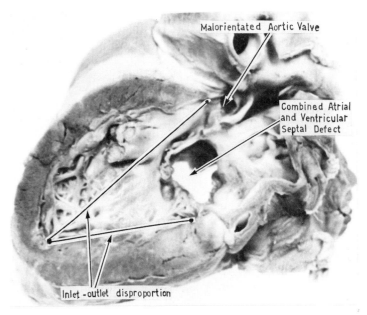

Malorientated Aortic Valve

Combined Atrial
and Ventricular
Septal Defect

Inlet-outlet disproportion

Fig. 20.2 A lateral view of the typical left ventricular morphology of an atrioventricular canal malformation. Note the marked disproportion between inlet and outlet lengths of the ventricle.

nosis of atrioventricular canal is exceedingly unlikely in the absence of a superior axis. *Echocardiography* can be diagnostic in that it may demonstrate a common atrioventricular valve passing 'through' the posterior interventricular septum (Fig. 9.15).

A step-up in oxygen saturation at atrial level is generally found at *cardiac catheterization*, indicating a left-to-right shunt. A further step-up at ventricular level would be expected, although this could reflect streaming through an atrial defect. Equal left and right ventricular pressures would be anticipated, and aortic and pulmonary systolic pressures will be the same. The diagnostic angiographic feature is the so-called 'goose-neck' deformity seen in the posterio-anterior projection of left ventricular angiography during diastole (Fig. 14.3). This is dependent partly upon abnormal anterior and rightward displacement of the aortic valve relative to the atrioventricular annulus and also to the abnormal orientation of this valve due to the disproportion of inlet (diaphragmatic) and outlet parts of the interventricular septum. This results in the inferior margin of the mitral component of the annulus being displaced downwards on the postero-anterior projection. Equally important is the irregularity of the left ventricular outflow tract seen during systole in the same projection. Outlined in diastole by undyed left atrial blood, a single atrioventricular valve orifice will be best demonstrated in the 'four chamber view' of Bargeron and Soto following left ventricular angiography. In this projection a 45° left anterior oblique tilt is coupled with a 45° craniocaudal tilt so that the posterior interventricular septum is seen in profile and the atrioventricular valve(s) are seen *en face*.

Treatment

Heart failure is treated with digoxin, diuretics, and potassium supplements. Surgical intervention is delayed as long as possible since corrective surgery is required on cardiopulmonary bypass. The necessity for fashioning two atrioventricular valves together with creation of new atrial and ventricular septa makes surgery technically difficult. There is little place for pulmonary artery banding as the left-to-right shunts are usually from left ventricle to right atrium (obligatory) (see p. 23).

Complex reconstruction of the cardiac anatomy is required. Frequently the bridging anterior leaflet has to be divided to form the septal leaflet of the tricuspid valve and part of the anterior cusp of the mitral valve. Since the lower atrial septum and upper ventricular septum are absent, a new atrioventricular septum must be reconstructed and attached to the existing septa, at the same time allowing re-attachment of the re-fashioned mitral and tricuspid valves. Damage to the abnormally placed atrioventricular node must be avoided. It is possible even in infants to correct this complex anomaly and produce competent mitral and tricuspid valves.

The hospital mortality for this complex form of congenital heart disease varies from 20–40 per cent.

References

Carpentier, A. (1978). Surgical anatomy and management of the mitral component of atrioventricular canal defects. In *Paediatric cardiology, 1977* (ed. R. H. Anderson and E. A. Shinebourne), pp. 477–86. Churchill Livingstone, Edinburgh.

Danielson, G. K. (1978). Correction of atrioventricular canal. In *Paediatric cardiology 1977* (ed. R. H. Anderson and E. A. Shinebourne), pp. 470–6. Churchill Livingstone, Edinburgh.

Feldt, R. H. (1976). *Atrioventricular canal defects*. W. B. Saunders, Philadelphia.

Rastelli, G. C., Kirklin, J. W., and Titus, J. L. (1966). Anatomic observations on complete form of persistent common atrioventricular canal with special reference to atrioventricular valves. *Mayo Clinic Proceedings* **41**, 296.

Van Mierop, L. H. S., Alley, R. D., Kausel, H. W., and Stranahan, A. (1962). The anatomy and embryology of endocardial cushion defects. *Journal of Thoracic and Cardiovascular Surgery* **43**, 71.

21 Ventricular septal defect (VSD)

Anatomy and embryology

As previously described, the ventricular septum is a complex structure (Fig. 21.1), having three muscular components (the inlet, trabecular, and outlet parts) and being completed by a fibrous component, the membranous septum (Fig. 21.1). Defects can exist either because the membranous septum does not close the interventricular communication, or because the muscular components themselves are improperly formed and fused. The reason why the membranous septum is unable to complete the septum is usually because of deficiency of the muscular components. These defects in the region of the membranous septum always have partly fibrous rims and are termed perimembranous (Figs. 21.2 and 21.3b). Another defect with a partially fibrous rim is the

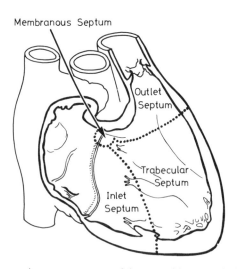

Fig. 21.1 The constituent components of the normal interventricular septum.

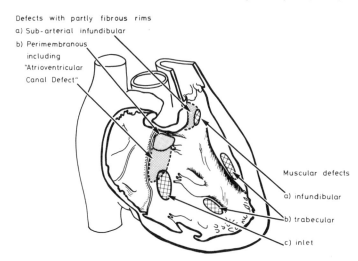

Defects with partly fibrous rims
a) Sub-arterial infundibular
b) Perimembranous
   including
   "Atrioventricular
   Canal Defect"

Muscular defects
a) infundibular
b) trabecular
c) inlet

Fig. 21.2 The relationship of ventricular septal defects to the constituent parts of the septum. Defects are divided into those with partly fibrous rims which may either be sub-arterial or perimembranous and those with entirely muscular rims. The muscular defects may be found in or between the infundibular trabecular or outlet components of the muscular septum.

sub-arterial infundibular defect. The fibrous tissue in this type is the fused aortic and pulmonary valves. This is the so-called 'supracristal' defect. The final type of defect is that with an entirely muscular rim. These muscular defects can be found in the inlet or infundibular septa or in the trabecular region towards the apex. Although these various defects are usually found in insolation, they may co-exist. The combination of multiple apical muscular defects may form a 'Swiss-cheese' type of septum. Because in the normal heart the aorta straddles the septum, but is closed off from the right ventricle by the membranous septum, in the presence of a perimembranous defect part of the aorta usually arises directly from the right ventricle (Fig. 21.4). This is termed aortic overriding. The degree of override varies, but is more marked when a perimembranous defect extends into the infundibular septum. In ventricular septal defects aortic override can occur until up to 50 per cent of the aorta is above the right ventricle. When more than 50 per cent aortic override occurs, the case would be considered a double outlet right ventricle. In infundibular defects, because of the lack of support for the aortic valve, prolapse of the right coronary cusp of the aortic valve is frequent with resultant aortic incompetence.

Distinguishing the type of defect is important with regard to the

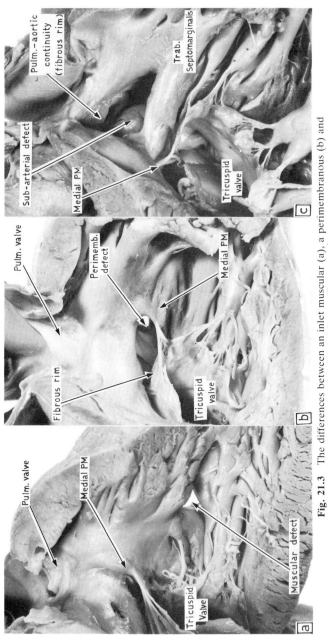

Fig. 21.3 The differences between an inlet muscular (a), a perimembranous (b) and a sub-arterial infundibular (c) defect. PM = papillary muscle.

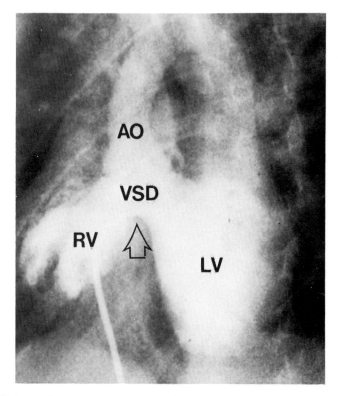

Fig. 21.4 Angiogram taken so as to profile the ventricular septum (open arrow) showing how the aorta (AO) overrides the cavity of the right ventricle (RV) in the presence of a perimembranous VSD. LV = left ventricle.

disposition of conduction tissue. In perimembranous defects the penetrating bundle is always in the postero-inferior rim, although its precise relationship to the edge of the defect varies considerably. In contrast, the bundle is supero-anterior to muscular defects in the inlet (between mitral and tricuspid valves) septum (Fig. 21.5). Because of this it is vital to distinguish an inlet (posterior) muscular defect from a perimembranous defect which extends into the inlet septum (so-called isolated atrioventricular canal type of defect). In this chapter only 'isolated' ventricular septal defects will be considered. Ventricular septal defects accompanying other malformations such as discordant or double outlet ventriculo-arterial connexions will be considered in their appropriate sections.

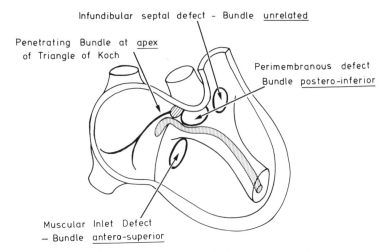

Fig. 21.5   The relationships of the atrioventricular bundle to various types of ventricular septal defect.

Incidence

The incidence of isolated ventricular septal defects shows a striking variation with age. In childhood it is the commonest congenital cardiac anomaly accounting for approximately 20 per cent of all malformations. In contrast, in adult life it is rare. The principal reason for this is that over 70 per cent of defects close spontaneously.

Clinical findings

Presentation

The symptomatology and clinical findings depend on the size of defect but are largely independent of its anatomical site. Small defects present as systolic murmurs in asymptomatic children. In contrast, large defects present in infancy, typically in the second month of life, with evidence of heart failure. Difficulty in feeding, dyspnoea, and chest infections are found. Failure to thrive, with the child falling below its percentiles for weight, also accompanies a large left-to-right shunt, although none of these features is specific for ventricular septal defects. As discussed previously (see p. 41), heart failure is dependent upon a large left-to-right shunt which occurs only when the high pulmonary vascular resistance present at birth has fallen. In rare cases (less than 5 per cent of large nonlimiting* defects) where resistance does not fall

*i.e. with a large enough defect so that right and left ventricular pressures are obligatorily equal.

postnatally or, alternatively, in older children when pulmonary vascular disease has progressed, the presenting feature may be intermittent cyanosis due to shunt reversal. Such children are usually below the third percentiles for height and weight.

Physical examination
The findings on physical examination depend on the size of defect, magnitude of shunt, and state of the pulmonary vascular resistance. With small shunts examination will be normal except for the characteristic pansystolic murmur (with or without thrill) maximal at the fourth or fifth left intercostal space at the sternal border. With larger shunts a mitral diastolic flow murmur will be heard (see Chapter 12) and as the pulmonary vascular resistance rises so the pulmonary component of the second sound becomes louder. In an out-patient clinic much time is or certainly should be spent in trying to determine if the second (pulmonary) component of the second sound is louder than the first component. Other findings on physical examination are not pathognomonic; with large shunts signs of heart failure and a chest bulge (from stiff lungs) may be present. Finally when the pulmonary vascular resistance is high the pulmonary component of the second sound becomes palpable.

The *chest X-ray* is normal with small defects. Cardiomegaly, left atrial enlargement and plethora (Fig. 7.1C) characterize larger defects. The aortic arch is almost always left-sided (with situs solitus and laevocardia), the presence of a right aortic arch strongly suggesting additional anomalies (i.e. tetralogy of Fallot). The *ECG* shows sinus rhythm and usually a normal P–R interval. The mean frontal QRS axis is usually normal although some large defects are associated with a superior axis. Tall P-waves in lead II (<3 mm) indicate right or left atrial hypertrophy. Evidence of right or biventricular hypertrophy is found in larger defects, right ventricular hypertrophy becoming marked as the pulmonary vascular resistance rises.

At *cardiac catheterization*, findings are dependent upon the size of the defect. In small defects, haemodynamic data may be normal and the defect detected only by angiography. With larger defects, right ventricular pressure rises until with large (non-limiting) defects, the ventricular pressures become equal. However, pulmonary artery diastolic and hence mean pressure will be lower than aortic. As the pulmonary vascular resistance rises so mean pulmonary arterial and aortic pressures will equalize. Oxygen saturation measurements will usually show a step-up in saturation at ventricular level, although this may disappear with rise in pulmonary vascular resistance. Angiograms in the left ventricle are mandatory and should be carried out using cineangiography in the projection best designed to profile the interventricular septum (see Chapter 7). 'The four chamber view' profiles the posterior (inlet) portion of the interventricular septum and the 'long axial' view the anterior part of the septum (Fig. 10.1b), thus allowing accurate assessment of both the siting and number of defects present. At catheterization it is imperative to exclude a ductus by aortography.

Treatment

Considerations of management must perforce take into account the natural history of the anomaly. As stated previously, 60 per cent of all defects seen in childhood will subsequently close. Thus all (small) defects without evidence of right ventricular hypertrophy require no therapy (except penicillin or penicillin and streptomycin prophylaxis for dental extractions), but should be followed up until the defect closes. Heart failure in infants with large defects should be treated with digoxin and diuretics. The indications for cardiac catheterization are as follows: persistence of cardiac failure or failure to thrive in infancy; the finding of a loud pulmonary component to the second sound, or increasing intensity of this sound, in particular when accompanied by electrocardiographic evidence of right ventricular hypertrophy*; ECG evidence of moderate to severe right ventricular hypertrophy*; recurrent chest infections especially if accompanied by evidence of lobar collapse; and finally, catheterization should be performed when the clinical diagnosis is uncertain in a symptomatic patient. As mentioned above, all sick infants should have arterial oxygen saturations measured in 100 per cent oxygen. Failure of arterial Po_2 to rise above 160 mm Hg in a patient thought to have a simple ventricular septal defect is thus also an indication for cardiac catheterization, as additional anomalies are probably present.

When cardiac catheterization has been performed, any child with a pulmonary artery pressure of less than half systemic should not be subjected to surgery, unless heart failure persists despite therapy. When pulmonary artery pressure is between half and two-thirds systemic, there is still a good chance for spontaneous closure and indications for surgery would be marked effort intolerance or persis-

---

*In our experience the single most useful indication for cardiac catheterization in a child with suspected ventricular septal defect is the finding of upright T waves in leads V_4R and V_1.

tent failure. With higher pulmonary artery pressures, the indications for surgery are stronger. In older children in this category, surgical closure should be performed. With children of under one year of age, surgical policies are still flexible. If there are multiple 'Swiss cheese' defects and the child is failing to thrive, pulmonary artery banding may be performed, especially in the first six months of life. When there is a single defect and failure, major paediatric cardiology units would probably advocate primary closure except in some infants under 4 kg when again pulmonary artery banding may be performed. Elective debanding and closure of residual defects can then be carried out after the age of one year. If the pulmonary vascular resistance is irreversibly elevated (see Chapter 4a) i.e. above eight units even with the patient breathing 100 per cent oxygen, then pulmonary vascular disease is present and surgery is contraindicated: the ventricular septal defect ensures that right ventricular pressure cannot rise above that in the left ventricle. If in the presence of severe pulmonary vascular disease the defect is closed, right ventricular pressure may rise precipitously and, even if the child survives operation, subsequent life expectancy would be shorter than without surgery.

Most defects can be closed via the right atrium and the tricuspid valve, thereby precluding the necessity for an incision in the right ventricle. The ventricular septal defect must be closed by means of a prosthetic patch (Dacron), or autologous tissue (pericardium) if preferred. Since there is an absolute deficiency in the ventricular septum causing the defect, it is not appropriate to close a ventricular septal defect by direct suture, which will almost certainly break away after the heart begins to contract. Even if it is not possible to close the ventricular septal defect through the transatrial route, visualization of the defect through the tricuspid valve allows accurate siting of the ventriculotomy. The hospital mortality for this condition is 0–5 per cent.

References

Hoffman, J. I. E. and Rudolph, A. M. (1965). The natural history of ventricular septal defect in infancy. *American Journal of Cardiology* **16**, 634.

Lincoln, C. (1978). Transatrial vs. ventricular closure of isolated ventricular septal defect. In *Paediatric cardiology, 1977* (ed. R. H. Anderson and E. A. Shinebourne), pp. 155–62. Churchill Livingstone, Edinburgh.

Moulaert, A. J. (1978). Anatomy of ventricular septal defect. In *Paediatric cardiology, 1977* (ed. R. H. Anderson and E. A. Shinebourne), pp. 113–124. Churchill Livingstone, Edinburgh.

Soto, B., Coghlan, C. H., and Bargeron, L. M. (1978). Angiography of ventricular septal defects. In *Paediatric cardiology, 1977* (ed. R. H. Anderson and E. A. Shinebourne), pp. 125–35. Churchill Livingstone, Edinburgh.

Turina, M. (1978). Early closure vs. two-stage treatment for ventricular septal defect. In *Paediatric cardiology, 1977* (ed. R. H. Anderson and E. A. Shinebourne), pp. 147–54. Churchill Livingstone, Edinburgh.

22 The univentricular heart (including absent AV connexion)

Nomenclature, anatomy, and embryology

Myriad terms have been used to describe the univentricular heart, including various definitions of the adjectives 'single' and 'common'. Categorization is dependent upon the definition of 'a ventricle'. We now define a ventricle as a chamber within the ventricular mass receiving one or more atrioventricular valves (inlet portions, Fig. 22.1). A chamber without such an inlet portion (or receiving less than half an atrioventricular valve) is defined as a rudimentary chamber. Rudimentary chambers can be of right or left ventricular type. They are termed outlet chambers if they give rise to (more than half) a great artery and trabecular pouches (of right or left ventricular pattern Fig. 22.1) when they do not. Thus trabecular pouches have neither inlet nor outlet valves. In a univentricular heart the atrioventricular inlet portions are dominantly committed to only one chamber in the ventricular mass, the ventricle while a rudimentary chamber may or may not be present. A univentricular heart exists either when both atrioventricular inlets (or more than half of any straddling inlet portions) drain to the same

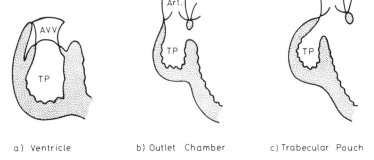

a) Ventricle   b) Outlet Chamber   c) Trabecular Pouch

Fig. 22.1 The components found in various types of ventricle and rudimentary chambers. AVV = atrioventricular valve; TP = trabecular portion; Art = artery.

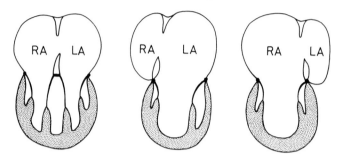

a) Double Inlet Ventricle   b) Absent Right AV Connexion   c) Absent Left AV Connexion

Fig. 22.2   The atrioventricular junctions found in double inlet ventricle and absence of the right or left atrioventricular connexion. RA = right atrium; LA = left atrium.

chamber (double inlet ventricle) or when one atrioventricular valve (inlet portion) is totally absent, as in the commonest form of a 'tricuspid atresia' (Fig. 22.2). We term the latter situation absence of one atrioventricular connexion (see Chapter 3).

Further subdivision of the univentricular heart (Fig. 22.3) is dependent upon the morphology of the chambers within the ventricular mass. By far the commonest variety has a main chamber with left ventricular trabecular pattern associated with a rudimentary chamber of right ventricular type. The rudimentary chamber is thought to be derived from the outlet portion of the primary heart tube together with the trabecular zone of right ventricular type which grows from this part of the primary tube (see Chapter 11). The septum separating the chambers is the trabecular septum and is an anterior structure, never

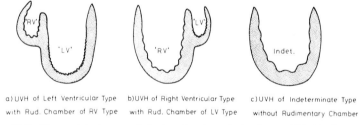

a) UVH of Left Ventricular Type   b) UVH of Right Ventricular Type   c) UVH of Indeterminate Type
   with Rud. Chamber of RV Type   with Rud. Chamber of LV Type   without Rudimentary Chamber

Fig. 22.3   The ventricular morphologies of univentricular hearts. NB: Rudimentary chambers may be right sided or left sided in either left ventricular or right ventricular varieties of univentricular heart. 'LV' = chamber of left ventricular morphology; 'RV' = chamber of right ventricular morphology; Indet. = chamber of indeterminate morphology.

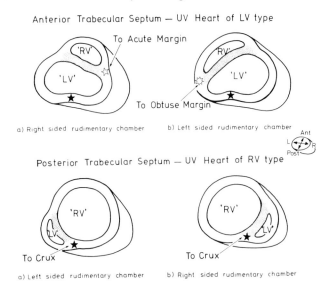

Fig. 22.4 The differences in septal orientation between univentricular (UV) hearts of left ventricular (LV) type and univentricular hearts of right ventricular (RV) type.

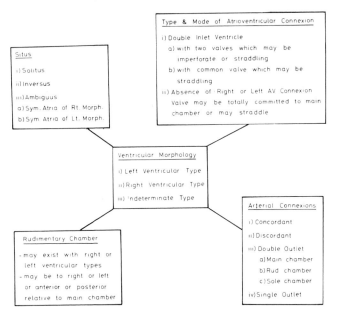

Fig. 22.5 The segmental approach to categorization of the univentricular heart.

extending to the crux of the heart (Fig. 22.4). This heart may be termed a univentricular heart of left ventricular type. Less common is the variety in which the inlet and outlet portions of the heart tube from an unseptated mass with coarse trabecular pattern—univentricular heart of indeterminate morphology without rudimentary chamber. A third variety of univentricular heart is that in which the valve-receiving chamber has right ventricular characteristics, with a posterior rudimentary chamber of left ventricular type. In these hearts the trabecular septum does extend to the crux cordis and is a posterior structure (Fig. 22.4). In univentricular hearts with rudimentary chambers arterial connexions may be concordant, discordant, double outlet, or single outlet. Use of concordance or discordance assumes that the nature of the trabecular zone of the outlet chamber as right or left ventricular in type can be ascertained. In contrast, in univentricular hearts without rudimentary chambers only double outlet or single outlet ventriculo-arterial connexions are possible (Fig. 22.5).

It is important to emphasize once more that absence of an atrioventricular connexion can exist with any ventricular morphology in a

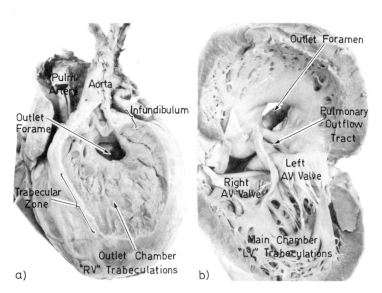

Fig. 22.6 The morphology of univentricular heart of left ventricular type with rudimentary chamber of right ventricular type. (a) shows the rudimentary chamber located on the left shoulder of the ventricular mass supporting a left sided aorta. (b) shows the main ventricular chamber which receives both atrioventricular valves and supports the pulmonary artery. The communication between the chambers is the outlet foramen.

univentricular heart. Thus the commonest form of tricuspid atresia is correctly described as univentricular heart of left ventricular type with absent right atrioventricular connexion. Similarly, some examples of 'mitral atresia' will be found with univentricular hearts. Furthermore, there may be variations in the mode of atrioventricular connexion. Thus, in double inlet ventricle, although both atria usually drain through separate atrioventricular valves they may also drain through a common valve; in addition one valve may straddle the trabecular septum providing that the degree of straddling results in less than 50 per cent of the valve connecting with the rudimentary chamber.

In practice, the commonest forms of univentricular heart are so-called 'single ventricle with outlet chamber' and so-called 'tricuspid atresia'. Both are univentricular hearts of left ventricular type, the former with double inlet and the latter with absent right atrioventricular connexion. Double inlet ventricle is most usually associated with arterial discordance, the aorta arising from a left-sided rudimentary chamber (Fig. 22.6). Less frequently the transposed aorta may arise from a right-sided rudimentary chamber and even more rarely the

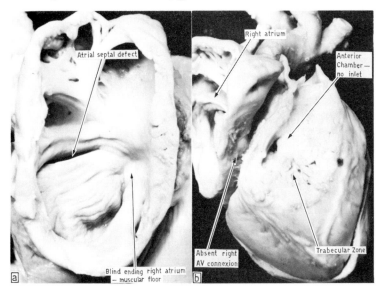

Fig. 22.7 The morphology of univentricular heart of left ventricular type with absent right atrioventricular connexions (tricuspid atresia). (a) shows the blind ending right atrium which contains no vestige of a tricuspid valve within its floor. (b) shows the rudimentary chamber of right ventricular type which is located on the right anterior shoulder of the ventricular mass. In this instance it supports the pulmonary artery (concordant ventriculo-arterial connexion).

pulmonary artery may arise from the rudimentary chamber and the aorta from the main chamber. The latter combination is frequently called the 'Holmes heart' (Fig. 22.12). A feature of these hearts is that, as in corrected transposition (see Chapter 28), the conduction tissue arises from an anterior node.. Tricuspid atresia is usually associated with concordant arterial connexions, and more rarely with arterial discordance (transposition). In the common form of tricuspid atresia, the tricuspid valve is totally absent, the right atrium having an entirely muscular floor (Fig. 22.7). Forms of tricuspid atresia with an imperforate tricuspid valve do exist, but are rare and are *not* univentricular. Although single ventricle and tricuspid atresia are the commonest forms, many other forms of univentricular heart exist, and sequential analysis is of particular value in diagnosing this malformation (Fig. 22.5).

Incidence

Although the anomaly is uncommon, increasing awareness of it facilitates its recognition. In the first year of life, it forms up to 10 per cent of symptomatic cyanotic heart disease.

Clinical findings

Presentation

Double inlet ventricle. As with the majority of complex cyanotic lesions, clinical presentation depends primarily on the effective pulmonary blood flow. With the commonly associated factor of pulmonary stenosis, cyanosis dominates the picture, and the patients fall into the group with cyanosis and pulmonary oligaemia on *chest X-ray* (see Chapter 7). In the absence of pulmonary outflow tract obstruction, heart failure with tachypnoea and hepatomegaly will be dominant. Cyanosis, if recognized, will be mild. Failure may be exacerbated by associated coarctation. These patients fall into the group of cyanosis with plethora on chest X-ray (see Chapter 7) and proof of the presence of cyanotic heart disease in these circumstances frequently depends upon blood gas analysis during administration of 100 per cent oxygen (see p. 36). If pulmonary stenosis is such that pulmonary flow is adequate but pulmonary hypertension absent, the patient may be so well compensated haemodynamically that there are no symptoms and the diagnosis may not be suspected until the second or third decade. *Absent right atrioventricular connexion—tricuspid atresia.* As already stated, the ventricular morphology found with 'tricuspid atresia' is as varied as with double inlet ventricles. Thus absence of the right atrioventricular connexion may be found with univentricular hearts of left, right, or indeterminate type. The ventriculo-arterial connexion may be concordant, discordant, double outlet, or single outlet. The commonest forms are in association with a univentricular heart of left ventricular type, rudimentary chamber of right ventricular type, and either concordant or discordant ventriculo-arterial connexions—corresponding to 'classical tricuspid atresia (Type I)' or to 'tricuspid atresia plus transposition of the great arteries (Type II)'. The former is usually associated with restricted pulmonary flow. The possible sites of obstruction alone or in combination are at the outlet foramen between main and outlet (rudimentary) chambers, within the outlet chamber itself, or at pulmonary valve level. Many of the patients with tricuspid atresia and discordant ventriculo-arterial connexions will have increased pulmonary flow, sometimes with coarctation (see Chapter 38) and rarely with subaortic stenosis.

Clinical presentation, as with double inlet ventricles, is dominated by the effect of associated anomalies on pulmonary flow.

Absent left atrioventricular connexion. When absent left atrioventricular connexion complicates the univentricular heart, extreme tachypnoea subsequent to pulmonary venous congestion (rates approximately 100 per minute) may be found, as the pulmonary venous return has to traverse the foramen ovale before reaching the ventricle.

Physical examination

Physical findings are in no way pathognomonic and depend largely on the associated anomalies. Arterial desaturation will always be present. In absent right atrioventricular connexion a prominent A-wave may be seen in the jugular venous pulse (see Chapter 6) which may be transmitted to the liver. With pulmonary stenosis an ejection systolic murmur will be heard; with pulmonary atresia there may be no murmurs and in both a single second sound is found. Conversely, with increased pulmonary flow the second sound is split with accentuation of the pulmonary component. The *chest X-ray* is non-specific but cardiomegaly is usually found. The *ECG* is extremely useful in differential diagnosis. Two main patterns are found. Dominant S waves across all the chest leads strongly suggest the diagnosis of double inlet ventricle of left ventricular type (Fig. 22.8). In contrast, the finding of signs of right atrial hypertrophy, a superior mean frontal QRS axis and left ventricular dominance would be indicative of univentricular heart of left ventricular type with absent right atrioventricular connexion (tricuspid atresia). (Fig. 22.9.) In any event, the presence of left ventricular dominance in a patient with cyanotic heart disease should raise the suspicion of univentricular heart of left ventricular type. The much less common univentricular heart of right ventricular type is characterized by right ventricular hypertrophy on ECG, a superior mean frontal QRS axis also being common as with all univentricular hearts.

Echocardiography (Chapter 9) is an invaluable tool in diagnosing this condition since absence of the inlet septum is easily detected. This feature is diagnostic of double inlet ventricle and is more readily established using echocardiography than with angiography. The technique almost always permits the number and nature of valves present to be determined. The finding of two valves obviously excludes the diagnosis of absent atrioventricular connexion. If a septum is found anterior to the valves, then the heart is of left ventricular type. In contrast, the finding of a septum posterior to two valves would be

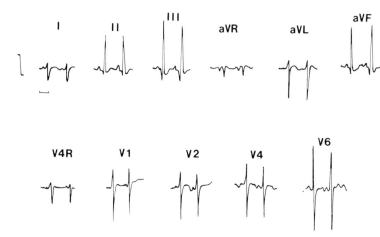

Fig. 22.8 ECG from a patient with univentricular heart of left ventricular type and double inlet. There are dominant S-waves across the horizontal chest leads (V1R, V6).

diagnostic of univentricular heart of right ventricular type with double inlet.

Cardiac catheterization in the presence of two atrioventricular valves will demonstrate a common mixing situation at ventricular level. There

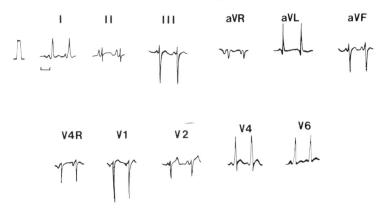

Fig. 22.9 ECG from a two-week-old patient with univentricular heart of left ventricular type and absent right atrioventricular connexion (tricuspid atresia). There is a superior mean frontal QRS axis of −35° with right atrial hypertrophy (P-wave of 3 mV in lead 2), and left ventricular dominance (dominant R-wave in V6 and S wave in V1).

will be admixture of systemic and pulmonary venous returns, usually giving similar saturations in both arteries. This may be modified by streaming effects. When there is absent right atrioventricular connexion (Fig. 22.10a) a right-to-left shunt at atrial level is encountered (a left-to-right shunt at atrial level excludes the diagnosis) while the converse applies for absent left atrioventricular connexion. Angiography will be required to define the ventricular anatomy (Fig. 22.10b), to demonstrate presence or absence of a rudimentary chamber (Fig. 22.11), and to determine the arterial connexion (Fig. 22.12). Atrial injections may also be required to define the atrioventricular connexions accurately (Fig. 22.10a).

Treatment
Treatment until recent years has been palliative. Pulmonary artery banding is performed when pulmonary flow is excessive, while systemic-pulmonary anastomoses are made for severely reduced pulmonary flow. In the last decade, more adventurous surgery has been attempted. In the absence of the right atrioventricular connexion, the right atrium has been connected directly to either the pulmonary artery or outlet chamber using homograft or prosthetic valve conduits (Fontan procedure). This approach has also been employed for double inlet ventricle after surgical closure of the right atrioventricular valve, providing the pulmonary artery pressure is low. Primary septation of the

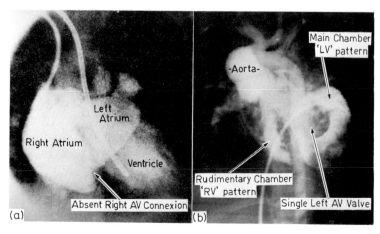

Fig. 22.10 Illustrative angiocardiograms from a patient with univentricular heart of left ventricular type and absent right atrioventricular connexion (tricuspid atresia). (a) shows a right atrial injection and illustrates that this chamber has no connexion either actual or potential with the ventricular mass. (b), from a different patient, illustrates an injection made in the ventricle and shows that this chamber has the characteristics of a left ventricle while the rudimentary chamber has right ventricular characteristics. There is only a single atrioventricular valve entering the ventricle.

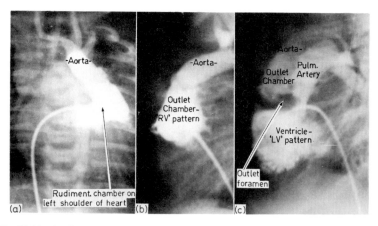

Fig. 22.11 Angiogram illustrating the chamber morphology in a univentricular heart of left ventricular type. (a) and (b) show the left-sided rudimentary chamber of right ventricular pattern in antero-posterior and lateral projections. The chamber supports the aorta (ventriculo-discordance). (c) shows the left ventricular main chamber giving rise to the pulmonary artery.

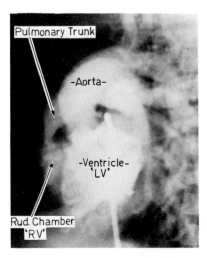

Fig. 22.12 Main chamber injection in a univentricular heart of left ventricular type showing the association with concordant arterial connexions. In other words the pulmonary trunk takes origin from the right ventricular rudimentary chamber and the aorta from the left ventricular main chamber.

univentricular heart with two atrioventricular valves has also been successfully performed. This technique carries a major risk of producing traumatic heart block owing to the unusual disposition of the atrioventricular conducting tissues in these hearts. Despite increasing knowledge of the anatomy, such operations are best carried out using intra-operative mapping techniques for identification of the bundle of His.

References

Anderson, R. H., Wilkinson, J. L., Gerlis, L. M., Smith, A., and Becker, A. E. (1977). Atresia of the right atrioventricular orifice. *British Heart Journal* **39**, 414.

Anderson, R. H., Wilkinson, J. L., and Becker, A. E. (1978). Conducting tissue in the univentricular heart. In *Embryology and tetralogy of the heart and the great arteries* (ed. L. H. S. Van Mierop, A. Oppenheimer-Dekker and C. Bruins), pp. 62–78. Boerhaave Series No. 13. Martinus Nijhoff. The Hague.

Anderson, R. H. and Shinebourne, E. A. (1978) Primitive ventricle. In *Paediatric cardiology, 1977* (ed. R. H. Anderson and E. A. Shinebourne), pp. 307–406. Churchill Livingstone, Edinburgh.

Van Praagh, R., Ongley, P. A., and Swan, H. J. C. (1964). Anatomic types of single or common ventricle in man. Morphologic and geometric aspects of 60 necropsied cases. *American Journal of Cardiology* **13**, 367.

23 Fallot's tetralogy

Anatomy and embryology

The four features of Fallot's tetralogy are ventricular septal defect, aortic overriding, pulmonary infundibular stenosis, and right ventricular hypertrophy. In anatomic terms, the tetralogy approximates to VSD with aortic overriding (see Chapter 21) except that in addition to the overriding, there is anterior deviation of the infundibular septum (Fig. 23.1). This deviation of the infundibular septum, increasing the diameter of the aorta at the expense of the pulmonary artery, contributes to pulmonary infundibular obstruction as do infundibular septal and infundibular wall hypertrophy. The right ventricular hypertrophy

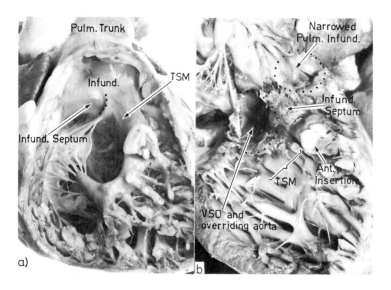

Fig. 23.1 The morphology of Fallot's tetralogy (b) compared with the normal heart (a). In the normal heart the anterior wall of the right ventricle has been cut away. Note how the infundibular septum inserts between the limbs of the trabecula septomarginalis (TSM) indicated by the dotted line. In Fallot's tetralogy the infundibular septum is inserted anterior to the trabecula septomarginalis producing at one and the same time a ventricular septal defect, an overriding aorta, and narrowing of the pulmonary infundibulum.

is a consequence of increased workload on the ventricle. The evidence of deviation of the infundibular septum is the placement of its septal insertion in front of the trabecula septomarginalis rather than between its limbs as is found in the normal heart (Fig. 23.1b) As may be anticipated, the precise anatomy of Fallot's tetralogy depends upon the degree of aortic overriding and septal deviation. Excessive anterior deviation results in pulmonary atresia with VSD. In contrast, minor degrees of deviation are indistinguishable from VSD with aortic overriding. In the latter cases, however, increasing hypertrophy may produce infundibular stenosis and result in 'classical' Fallot's tetralogy. The degree of aortic overriding may similarly be minimal or extreme. When the aortic override is such as to place more than half the aorta above the right ventricle, the case by definition would be considered as double outlet right ventricle (see Chapter 3). It should be stressed that the infundibular anatomy described is an essential part of Fallot's tetralogy. VSD with aorta overriding and pulmonary *valvar* stenosis should not be defined as Fallot's tetralogy.

Incidence
The lesion is common, accounting for approximately 10 per cent of all congenital cardiac anomalies.

Clinical findings

Presentation
The mode of presentation and age at presentation are both dependent on the severity of pulmonary outflow tract obstruction. When obstruction is severe at birth, the child presents as a neonatal emergency with profound cyanosis . At the other extreme, when infundibular obstruction is negligible, the infant presents with heart failure at 2–3 months of age and evidence of a left-to-right shunt. More commonly a systolic murmur is heard in an otherwise asymptomatic child but cyanosis develops during the first year. This reflects increasing infundibular obstruction. A further group of patients present with episodic unconsciousness and cyanosis due to infundibular spasm.

The degree of cyanosis present is dependent upon the severity of right ventricular outflow tract obstruction. When this is moderate to severe, the child is blue at rest and exhibits finger clubbing. Pulses are normal but a prominent parasternal (right ventricular) impulse is felt. The first heart sound is normal, the second single, and an ejection systolic murmur is audible, maximal at the left sternal border in the third intercostal space. An aortic ejection click may be present, reflecting the large size of the ascending aorta.

Physical examination

Chest *X-ray* shows normal heart size with a pulmonary artery 'bay', which is a consequence of diminution in size of the main pulmonary artery. The lung fields are oligaemic, the reduction in pulmonary vascular markings being dependent on the degree of infundibular obstruction. A right aortic arch is present in 20 per cent of cases (Fig. 7. 1). The X-ray finding of a right arch with oligaemic lung fields is strongly suggestive of Fallot's tetralogy or pulmonary atresia with ventricular septal defect. Acyanotic Fallot's tetralogy should always be considered in a child with signs of a ventricular septal defect when a right arch accompanies normal vascular markings. The *ECG* shows sinus rhythm with a normal P–R interval. Peaked P-waves in lead 2 may be present, indicative of right atrial hypertrophy, and there is usually evidence of right ventricular hypertrophy. Right axis deviation is found, with the axis varying between $+80°$ and $+160°$. A superior axis in a patient with findings compatible with Fallot's tetralogy would be suggestive of double outlet right ventricle with pulmonary stenosis, but is occasionally found in Fallot's tetralogy with concordant ventriculo-arterial connexions.

Findings at *cardiac catheterization* are dependent upon the severity of outflow tract obstruction. There is a right-to-left shunt at ventricular level, although frequently this shunt is only detected at aortic level. Ventricular pressures are equal as the defect is always large. If outflow tract obstruction is minimal, a left-to-right shunt may be detected at initial catheterization. The shunt subsequently reverses as a consequence of increasing obstruction. *Angiocardiography* is optimally performed in right and left ventricles, and the aorta. Right ventriculography demonstrates a normally connected pulmonary artery with aortic filling through a ventricular septal defect. In deeply cyanosed neonates not only is outflow tract obstruction severe but the pulmonary arteries may be very small (Fig. 23.2). More commonly, and particularly in older children, infundibular stenosis marked during systole (Fig. 23.3) but minimal during diastole is seen, with larger pulmonary arteries. Additional valvar stenosis may be present (Fig. 23.4), although the latter is not an essential feature of tetralogy. Aortic-mitral valve continuity is usually demonstrated by left ventriculography as will be the degree of aortic override and the precise anatomy of the ventricular septal defect. Aortography should be

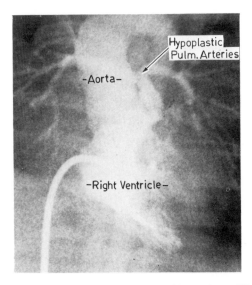

Fig. 23.2 Right ventricular angiogram in neonate with tetralogy of Fallot and severe pulmonary outflow tract obstruction. The projection is the four chamber view of Bargeron and Soto. The pulmonary arteries are extremely hypoplastic, the diameter of the main pulmonary artery being less than one-fifth that of the ascending aorta. Primary correction is not possible in such patients.

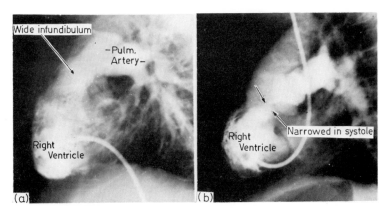

Fig. 23.3 Right ventriculogram in patient with tetralogy of Fallot. (a) indicates diastole and shows a widely dilated right ventricular outflow tract. During systole (b) marked infundibular narrowing is seen (indicated by arrows) while the pulmonary valve anulus and pulmonary valve appear normal. Prolonged infundibular shut-down produces hypercyanotic attacks.

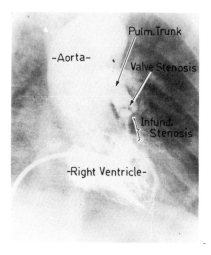

Fig. 23.4   Right ventriculogram in frontal projection in a patient with severe tetralogy of Fallot. In addition to severe infundibular stenosis there is valvar pulmonary stenosis and a small pulmonary valve anulus.

performed in order to determine the presence or absence of a persistent ductus or systemic–pulmonary collateral arteries.

Treatment

In the first few months of life, if cyanosis is severe, a surgical systemic – pulmonary anastomosis may be performed between the back of the aorta and the front of the right pulmonary artery (Waterston shunt) although in all infants, when a shunt is deemed necessary, a Blalock – Taussig shunt between right subclavian and right pulmonary artery would be preferred. When the arch is right-sided, a left-sided Blalock – Taussig anastomosis would be performed. Hypercyanotic attacks due to infundibular shutdown are treated by oxygen administration, correction of acidosis, and a β-adrenergic blocking agent such as propranolol (0.1 mg/kg). If a child over the age of one year is persistently blue, total correction on cardiopulmonary bypass should be undertaken. The decision to attempt total correction in young infants and children is dependent upon the anatomy of the main right and left pulmonary arteries. If these vessels are hypoplastic—that is, less than one-third the diameter of the aorta (Fig. 23.2)—and if the patient is under 5 kg in weight, the results of palliation are generally superior to those of total correction. Under these circumstances one further surgical approach is to relieve the outflow tract obstruction on cardiopulmonary bypass but to leave the ventricular septal defect: a technique that gives the best chance of subsequent growth of the pulmonary arteries.

Successful intracardiac repair of tetralogy of Fallot is dependent on closure of the ventricular septal defect(s), relief of right ventricular outflow tract obstruction at ventricular, pulmonary valve, and pulmonary artery levels, and preservation of the myocardium from prolonged ischaemia or damage to the coronary arteries.

When the main pulmonary artery and pulmonary valve ring are small, it is often necessary to enlarge them by means of a gusset. Similarly when marked anterior displacement of the infundibular septum is the cause of outflow tract obstruction a gusset is also placed in the right ventriculotomy. The ventricular septal defect is closed by means of a prosthetic patch (Dacron). Since the placement of this patch is in the region of the atrioventricular conducting tissue, knowledge of its distribution is obligatory for surgical closure, as damage can result in atrioventricular dissociation. In 2 per cent of patients the anterior descending coronary artery is supplied by a large branch from the right coronary artery, which crosses the right ventricular outflow tract. In this case, obstruction to outflow from the right ventricle into the pulmonary artery must be relieved by means of an external tube conduit, since division of this anomalous artery would cause fatal ischaemia of the left ventricle.

The result of treatment in this condition is 1–8 per cent mortality in children and around 10–15 per cent in infants.

References

Bargeron, L. M., Elliot, L. P., Soto, B., Bream, P. R., and Curry, G. C. (1977). Axial angiocardiography in congenital heart disease. Technical and anatomical considerations. *Circulation* **56**, 1075.

Becker, A. E., Connor, M., and Anderson, R. H. (1975). Tetralogy of Fallot: a morphometric and geometric study. *American Journal of Cardiology* **35**, 402.

Goor, D. A., Lillehei, C. W., and Edwards, J. E. (1971). Ventricular septal defects and pulmonic stenosis with and without dextroposition. Anatomic features and embryologic implications. *Chest* **60**, 117.

Honey, M., Chamberlain, D. A., and Howard, J. (1964). The effect of beta-sympathetic blockade on arterial oxygen saturation in Fallot's tetralogy. *Circulation* **30**, 501.

Kirklin, J. W. and Karp, R. (1970). *The tetralogy of Fallot: from a surgical viewpoint.* W. D. Saunders, New York.

Pacifico, A. D., Bargeron, L. M., and Kirklin, J. W. (1973). Primary total correction of tetralogy of Fallot in children less than four years of age. *Circulation* **48**, 1085.

Shinebourne, E. A., Anderson, R. H. and Bowyer, J. J. (1975). Variations in clinical presentation of Fallot's tetralogy in infancy. *British Heart Journal* **37**, 946.

Wood, P. (1958). Attacks of deeper cyanosis and loss of consciousness (syncope) in Fallot's tetralogy. *British Heart Journal* **20**, 282.

24 Pulmonary atresia with intact interventricular septum

The nature of pulmonary atresia depends on the attachment of the atretic pulmonary trunk and the ventricular origin of the aorta. However, whatever the ventricular origin of the great arteries pulmonary atresia can exist in two distinct forms: first, with an intact ventricular septum, and secondly, with a ventricular septal defect. The clinical problems posed by the two conditions are entirely different and they will, therefore, be considered separately.

Anatomy and embryology
In the commonest form of pulmonary atresia with intact septum the pulmonary remnant is attached to the right ventricle and the aorta arises from the left ventricle. The obstruction to right ventricular outflow can be predominantly at infundibular level or at pulmonary valve level (Fig. 24.1). In the former case there may be up to 10 mm between the blind end of the right ventricle and the patent proximal pulmonary artery. The right ventricular cavity is usually grossly reduced but may rarely be dilated. The tricuspid valve is usually dysplastic and frequently exhibits Ebstein's malformation. The right ventricular myocardium is hypertrophied and may be cavitated by sinusoids which drain retrogradely from the cavity to the coronary arteries (Fig. 24.2). Tricuspid incompetence is not uncommon together with right atrial enlargement. The main exit for right-sided blood is through the foramen ovale. Pulmonary blood flow occurs from the aorta through a persistent ductus arteriosus. The main and proximal portions of the right and left pulmonary arteries are present. Pulmonary atresia with intact septum and the aorta arising from the right ventricle is a much rarer anomaly. It is a variant of complete transposition (see Chapter 27).

Incidence
Pulmonary atresia with intact septum is one of the commonest causes of severe cyanosis in the neonatal period, but is rarely seen beyond this age if untreated as most patients die as neonates.

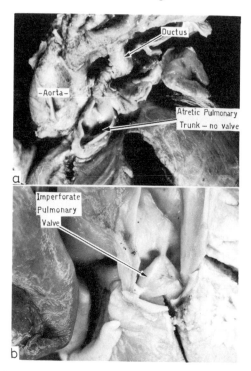

Fig. 24.1 The different types of pulmonary trunk morphology found in patients with pulmonary atresia with intact interventricular septum. (a) shows the opened atretic pulmonary trunk from a patient with infundibular atresia. There is no valve tissue to be seen. Note that the pulmonary supply is via a ductus; (b), in contrast, shows a patient with an imperforate pulmonary valve between pulmonary trunk and the right ventricle. This patient is much more amenable to corrective procedures.

Clinical findings

It is usual for presentation to occur in the first week of life with intense cyanosis. On examination there is a single second sound usually with no significant murmurs. Profound pulmonary oligaemia is observed on the *chest X-ray* with a left aortic arch and a concave pulmonary bay in the cardiac silhouette. Cardiomegaly may be present depending on the degree of right atrial enlargement. The major *ECG* feature is of a paucity of right-sided ventricular forces with left ventricular dominance, i.e. adult pattern. There may be right atrial hypertrophy and the mean frontal (QRS) axis is normal. At *cardiac catheterization* it will prove impossible to enter the pulmonary artery from the right ventricle but the catheter can easily be passed to the left atrium. There is a

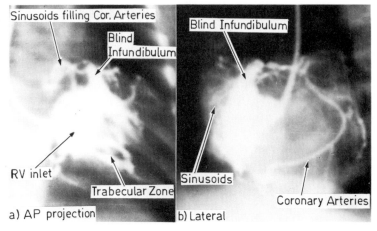

Fig. 24.2 Right ventriculogram in patient with pulmonary atresia and intact interventricular septum. In the frontal projection (a) the right ventricle is seen to have an extremely small cavity but thick wall. Both in this projection and in (b) the lateral projection, retrograde filling of the coronary arterial tree takes place via coronary sinusoids.

right-to-left shunt at atrial level and arterial desaturation. The right ventricular pressure is typically above systemic pressure. Angiography confirms the diagnosis (Fig. 24.2) and will distinguish pulmonary atresia from critical pulmonary stenosis.

Treatment
There is considerable debate at the present time as to the optimal treatment of this condition. There are two problems: the first is to achieve adequate pulmonary flow as an emergency procedure to sustain life and the second is to establish antegrade flow from right ventricle to pulmonary artery in the hope that both will grow. Palliation can be achieved by the combination of a systemic-pulmonary shunt with or without atrial septostomy or septectomy. Even more rapid short-term palliation can be achieved by infusion of prostaglandin E_1 or E_2 (0.05 μg/kg body weight/minute) which dilates the ductus arteriosus hence increasing pulmonary flow. The problem remains, however, as to what if anything can be done to encourage growth of the right ventricle. Certainly valvotomy alone nearly always ends with the death of the infant. Some surgeons perform an open or closed pulmonary valvotomy within one month of a shunt, but later corrective surgery after these two procedures has been only sporadically successful. Many units now are advocating a Fontan type of

procedure (valved conduit from right atrium to main pulmonary artery) as an alternative approach, while others would suggest that the generally bad prognosis of the anomaly should perhaps be a reason not even to palliate.

References

Bowman, F. O., Malm, J. R., Hayer, C. J., Gersony, W. M., and Ellis, K. (1976) Pulmonary atresia with intact ventricular septum. *Journal of Thoracic and Cardiovascular Surgery* **37**, 124.

Freedom, R. M. and Keith, J. D. (1978). Pulmonary atresia with normal aortic root. In *Heart disease in infancy and childhood.* (ed. J. D. Keith, R. D. Rowe, and P. Vlad), pp. 506–17. Macmillan, New York.

Miller, G. A. H., Restifo, M., Shinebourne, E. A., Paneth, M., Joseph, M. C., Lennox, S. C., and Kerr, I. H. (1973). Pulmonary atresia with intact ventricular septum and critical pulmonary stenosis presenting in the first month of life. Investigation and surgical results. *British Heart Journal* **35**, 9.

Zuberbuhler, J. R. and Anderson, R. H. (1979). Morphological variations in pulmonary atresia with intact ventricular septum. *British Heart Journal.* **41**, 281.

25 Pulmonary atresia with ventricular septal defect

Anatomy and embryology

The precise anatomy of pulmonary atresia in the presence of a ventricular septal defect depends upon the ventricular origin of the aorta, the relationship of the aorta to the pulmonary artery remnant, if present, and the source of the pulmonary blood supply. In the commonest form of the anomaly the atretic pulmonary trunk is attached to

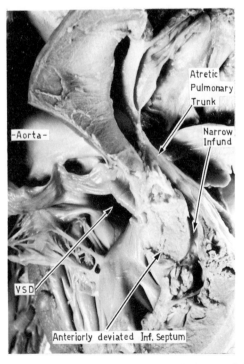

Fig. 25.1 A specimen of pulmonary atresia with ventricular septal defect which has been dissected to illustrate the origin of the aorta from the right ventricle overriding a ventricular septal defect and the potential connexion between the atretic pulmonary trunk and the blind ending right ventricular infundibulum. Note the anterior deviation of the infundibular septum. Compare with **Fig. 23.1**.

the right ventricular infundibulum and the aorta overrides the ventricular septal defect (Fig. 25.1) Developmentally this situation can be considered as tetralogy of Fallot with pulmonary atresia due to excessive anterior deviation of the infundibular septum (Compare Fig. 25.1 and 23.1a). This variety is then further divided depending on the source of pulmonary blood flow, and the presence or absence of the main right and left pulmonary arteries. The intrapulmonary arteries form *in situ*. The arteries supplying these are either the ductus arteriosus (Fig. 25.2), small broncho-pulmonary anastomoses, or large systemic-pulmonary collateral vessels (Fig. 25.3). In the first two cases, main, right, and left pulmonary arteries are normally present; in the last, they may be absent ('absent sixth arch'). When present the true right and left pulmonary arteries may be confluent or non-confluent. The blood supply to the intrapulmonary vessels may be unifocal or multifocal. In the latter case, even if the main right and left pulmonary arteries are present they may not link up with all the intrapulmonary

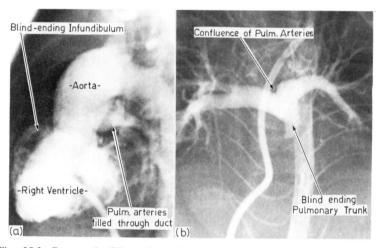

Fig. 25.2 Retrograde filling of small pulmonary arteries via persistent ductus arteriosus in patient with pulmonary atresia and ventricular septal defect.

vessels. In rarer instances the atretic pulmonary artery remnant may be posterior to the aorta, which arises entirely from the right ventricle, and be directed towards the left ventricle. This anomaly can be considered as complete transposition with pulmonary atresia and ventricular septal defect. As with the 'tetralogy' variant, the source of pulmonary blood supply is variable and forms the basis for further subdivision.

Incidence
It is a relatively uncommon cause of cyanotic heart disease.

Clinical findings
Presentation depends mainly on the magnitude of the pulmonary blood flow. Thus profound cyanosis in the neonatal period will be found in those with flow derived solely from a closing ductus. In contrast, some asymptomatic adults with this condition are diagnosed when a continuous murmur is heard during incidental examination, cyanosis being barely detectable clinically. The murmur is due to flow through large systemic pulmonary collateral arteries which are often tortuous and stenosed at their junction with the intrapulmonary vasculature (Fig. 25.3). These patients have a balanced haemodynamic situation where pulmonary flow is optimal (cf. univentricular heart, Chapter 22). At auscultation there will be a single second sound and either a continuous murmur or sometimes no murmurs. In older chil-

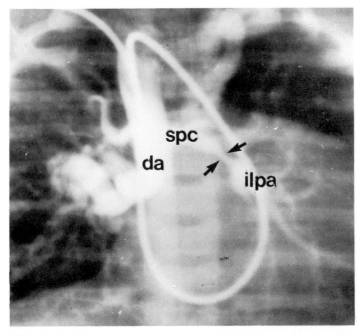

Fig. 25.3 Descending aortogram (frontal projection) from a patient with pulmonary atresia and ventricular septal defect, systemic pulmonary collaterals (spc) arising from the descending aorta (da) supply the intra-lobar pulmonary arteries (ilpa). The stenosis (arrowed) marks the junction between the superior vena cava (svc) and the intra-lobar pulmonary arteries.

dren, lack of a murmur may be the distinguishing clinical feature from Fallot's tetralogy.

Physical examination

On *chest X-ray* the pulmonary vascular markings depend on the magnitude of flow, varying from oligaemia through normality to plethora with abnormal vascular markings. Heart size is usually normal. Hypoplasia of the main pulmonary artery produces a 'bay' in the cardiac silhouette and a right aortic arch is seen in approximately 30 per cent of cases. *ECG* normally exhibits right atrial and definite right ventricular hypertrophy (cf. pulmonary atresia with intact septum). The mean frontal QRS axis is to the right or normal. *Cardiac catheterization* reveals right-to-left or even bidirectional shunting at ventricular level. There will be arterial desaturation and a pulmonary artery will not be entered. Right ventricular angiography and aortography are required

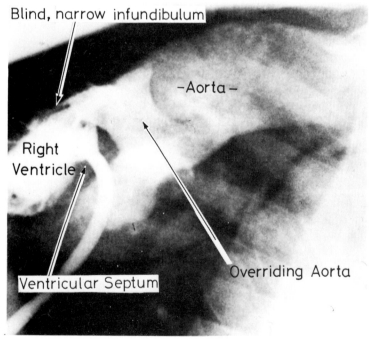

Fig. 25.4 Right ventricular angiogram in a patient with pulmonary atresia and ventricular septal defect. Overriding of the aorta is clearly demonstrated as is the blind ending infundibulum.

to confirm the diagnosis (Fig. 25.4). Selective injections into collateral arteries are necessary to define the precise pulmonary vascular supply, and also to demonstrate by retrograde filling whether confluent right and left pulmonary arteries are present.

Treatment

When the defects amount to an extreme form of tetralogy of Fallot, palliation by systemic pulmonary anastomosis is performed early in life, with total correction after the age of five years. In the smaller group with no true pulmonary arteries total correction is not possible, although palliative shunts can again improve symptoms. The shunts are performed both to increase pulmonary blood flow and to encourage growth of the pulmonary vascular bed.

In later life, total correction can be carried out along the same principles as that of correction of tetralogy of Fallot; that is, the ventricular septal defect is closed and right ventricular-pulmonary artery continuity is re-established. It is nearly always necessary to re-connect the right ventricle to the confluence of right and left pulmonary arteries by means of an external valved conduit. There are frequently very large systemic artery/pulmonary artery collateral vessels present, which must be ligated before corrective surgery is performed. Failure to ligate these large vessels can result in high output cardiac failure which increases the post-operative morbidity.

The hospital mortality for 'corrective' surgery is still 20 per cent to 35 per cent even when reasonable-sized sixth arch structures are present.

References

Macartney, F. J., Deverall, P. B., and Scott, O. (1973). Haemodynamic characteristics of systemic arterial blood supply to the lungs. *British Heart Journal* **35**, 28.

Macartney, F. J., Scott, O., and Deverall, P. B. (1974). Haemodynamic and anatomical characteristics of pulmonary blood supply in pulmonary atresia with ventricular septal defect—including a case of persistent fifth aortic arch. *British Heart Journal* **36**, 1049.

Ross, D. N. and Somerville, J. (1966). Correction of pulmonary atresia with homograft aortic valve. *Lancet* **2**, 1446.

Thiene, G., Bortolotti, U., Gallucci, V., Valente, M. L., and Dalla Volta, S. (1977). Pulmonary atresia with ventricular septal defect. *British Heart Journal* **39**, 1223.

26 Hypoplastic left heart syndrome

Anatomy and embryology

Hypoplastic left heart syndrome describes the constellation of anomalies characterized by aortic atresia and hypoplasia of the left heart chambers. Almost always the great arteries are normally related, but the aortic root is devoid of valve tissue, being a blind-ending diverticulum beneath the level of the coronary arteries (Fig. 26.1). The

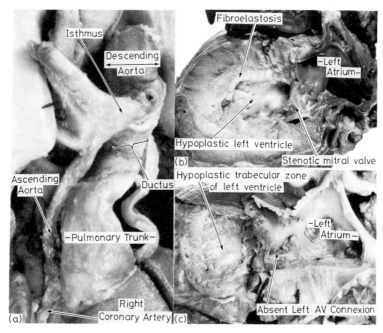

Fig. 26.1 (a) Photograph of a heart with aortic atresia and hypoplasia of the left-sided chambers showing the great arteries. The aorta is blind ending and gives rise to the coronary arteries. It is filled in retrograde fashion from a ductus arteriosus which also supplies the descending aorta. (b) and (c) the different ventricular morphologies found in hypoplastic left heart syndrome. (b) shows a hypoplastic left ventricle in a patient with severe mitral stenosis and fibroelastosis while (c) shows the rudimentary chamber of left ventricular type in a patient with absence of the left atrioventricular connexion.

arch expands from a narrow cord at the base of the heart to the arch, but none the less the arch is considerably smaller than the pulmonary artery. The lower body receives blood from the pulmonary trunk via a persistent ductus and the head and neck arteries receive the same stream via the isthmus, which frequently shows additional localized coarctation. The ascending aorta conducts blood to the coronary arteries in retrograde fashion. Two basic morphologies of the left ventricle are found with aortic atresia. In one the left atrioventricular connexion is absent and the left ventricular chamber is rudimentary, represented only by its trabecular component (Fig. 26.1b). This is a variety of univentricular heart (see Chapter 22). In the other and much commoner form, with concordant atrioventricular connexions, the mitral valve is formed but grossly stenosed, and the left ventricular cavity usually exhibits severe fibro-elastosis (Fig. 26.1c). In both types the ventricular septum is intact. In rare instances the left ventricle and mitral valve may be of good size when associated with severe aortic atresia because of an accompanying ventricular septal defect. The hypoplastic left heart syndrome results from inadequate flow through the left heart during fetal development and may be consequent upon stenosis or atresia at the aortic valve, mitral valve, or foramen ovale.

Incidence
It is one of the commonest causes of death due to congenital heart disease in the first week of life.

Clinical findings
Presentation is usually in the first week of life. The infant is severely ill, grey, shocked, and tachypnoeic. Signs of heart failure are present and the pulses are exceedingly weak, with the lower limb pulses being more easily palpable than upper limb pulses (cf. coarctation). The blood pressure is low. Cyanosis may be difficult to detect clinically although arterial desaturation is present as revealed by blood gas analysis following 100 per cent oxygen administration. Arterial blood analysis will also demonstrate a severe metabolic acidosis reflecting poor tissue perfusion. On auscultation the second heart sound is single and loud. There may be no murmurs.

Chest X-ray shows pulmonary venous congestion or even frank oedema. The aortic knuckle is absent and there may be cardiomegaly. *ECG* shows a paucity of left ventricular forces, but the right ventricular dominance may not be inappropriate for the age of the patient. A superior mean frontal QRS axis is sometimes found. *Echocardiogra-*

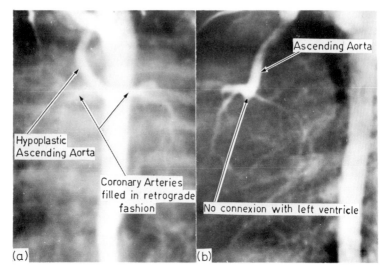

Fig. 26.2 (a) Aortogram demonstrating the severely hypoplastic ascending aorta through which the coronary vessels are supplied in retrograde fashion. This contrasts with the normal size of descending aorta (b).

phy will demonstrate a minute posterior ventricular chamber as well as hypoplasia of the posterior great artery (Fig. 9.6). The echocardiogram may be diagnostic, and hence, in conjunction with the clinical findings, may obviate the need for formal cardiac catheterization. Should *catheterization* be performed, a low arterial blood pressure is found. There will be a left-to-right shunt at atrial level, the right ventricle will be at systemic pressure, and the descending aorta is entered from the right heart via a ductus. Angiography confirms the diagnosis, the essential feature being the minute size of the ascending aorta (Fig. 26.2).

Treatment
At the time of writing there is no treatment for this condition. However, reconstructive surgery may be feasible for those rare cases of aortic atresia with good-sized left ventricles.

References
Doty, D. B. and Knott, H. W. (1977). Hypoplastic left heart syndrome. Experience with an operation to establish functionally normal circulation. *Journal of Thoracic and Cardiovascular Surgery* **74**, 624.

Freedom, R. M., Culham, J. A. G., Moes, C. A. F., and Harrington, D. (1976). Selective aortic root angiography in the hypoplastic left heart syndrome. *European Journal of Cardiology* **4**, 25.

Krovetz, L. J., Rowe, R. D., and Scheibler, G. L. (1970). Hemodynamics of aortic valve atresia. *Circulation* **42**, 953.

Pellegrino, P. A. and Thiene, G. (1976). Aortic valve atresia with a normally developed left ventricle. *Chest* **65**, 1.

27 Complete transposition

Definition
The term transposition of the great arteries describes only the connexion of ventriculo-arterial discordance in which the aorta arises from the morphologically right ventricle and the pulmonary artery from the morphologically left ventricle. Thus both great arteries arise from morphologically inappropriate ventricles. As indicated in the section on sequential chamber localization, full segmental description of any heart with abnormal connexions is desirable. However, transposition itself is qualified by the terms 'physiologically complete or corrected' depending on the atrioventricular connexion.

Complete transposition assumes the presence of atrioventricular concordance so that the systemic venous return is directed to the aorta.

Corrected transposition assumes atrioventricular discordance so that systemic venous return is distributed to the lungs, albeit by the morphologically left ventricle.

COMPLETE TRANSPOSITION WITH OR WITHOUT VENTRICULAR SEPTAL DEFECT

Anatomy and embryology
Complete transposition, the commonest form of transposition of the great arteries, is the combination of situs solitus, atrioventricular concordance, and ventriculo-arterial discordance. The blood passes from the right atrium to the right ventricle and thence to the aorta (Fig. 27. 1a). Pulmonary venous return is directed from left atrium through the left ventricle to the pulmonary artery (Fig. 27.1b). For survival a communication between the systemic and pulmonary circuits is essential. This may be at atrial, ventricular, or ductal level. The typical anatomy in transposition is for the aortic valve to be completely supported by muscle (the infundibulum of the right ventricle) while the pulmonary valve is in fibrous continuity with the mitral valve. Usually the aortic valve is to the right of the pulmonary valve. Less frequently

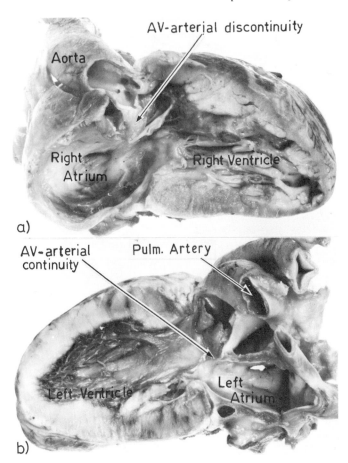

Fig. 27.1   A specimen of complete transposition (situs solitus, atrioventricular concordance, ventriculo-arterial discordance) dissected to show the difference between the right- and left-sided heart chambers. (a) shows the right atrium communicating with the right ventricle via the tricuspid valve, the right ventricle supporting the aorta. There is discontinuity between the atrioventricular (AV) and the arterial valves. (b) shows the left-sided chambers. The left atrium communicates with the left ventricle through the mitral valve, the left ventricle supporting the pulmonary artery. There is continuity between the pulmonary and mitral valves.

the aortic valve may be to the left of the pulmonary valve, or occasionally directly in front. In rare instances the aortic valve may be posterior to the pulmonary valve. Thus spatial relationships are of little importance when making the diagnosis of ventriculo-arterial discordance. Transposition can co-exist with anomalies of any of the cardiac

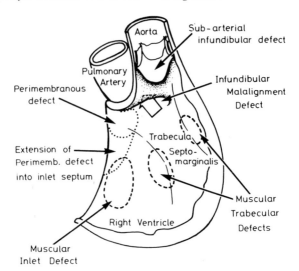

Fig. 27.2 The varieties of ventricular septal defect which may be encountered in patients with complete transposition.

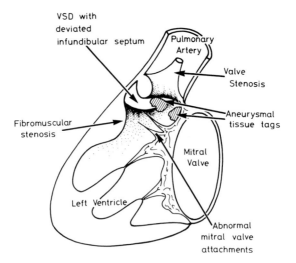

Fig. 27.3 The types of pulmonary outflow tract stenosis which may be encountered in patients with complete transposition.

segments. Of particular importance are the associations with ventricular septal defect, which may exist in various parts of the septum (Fig. 27.2), persistent ductus arteriosus and pulmonary stenosis (Fig. 27.3). Pulmonary atresia can also be present when the aorta arises in its entirety from the right ventricle. In specimens it is usually possible to trace the atretic pulmonary trunk to the left ventricle, and that combination can then be justifiably termed complete transposition with pulmonary atresia. It can exist with or without a ventricular septal defect, as can pulmonary atresia with normally connected arteries (see Chapters 24 and 25). In a clinical situation, however, it may not be possible to ascertain the ventricular origin of the atretic pulmonary trunk. Single outlet of the heart is then a more accurate description. Transposition is also often found in association with univentricular hearts of left ventricular type with either double inlet or absence of the right atrioventricular connexion (see Chapter 22).

The mode of development of ventriculo-arterial discordance is controversial. It has generally been held that the ventricular origins of the great arteries are reversed following development of a straight, rather than spiral, infundibulo-truncal septum. Considerable evidence has accrued recently to show that transposition may result from transfer of the pulmonary artery instead of the aorta from the outlet zone of the heart tube to the left ventricle. Thus it may result from infundibular maldevelopment, whereby the sub-pulmonary rather than sub-aortic infundibulum is absorbed, or a combination of both infundibular maldevelopment and truncal malseptation.

Incidence

Complete transposition is the commonest cause of cyanotic congenital heart disease in the first month of life, accounting for at least 25 per cent of all such patients.

Clinical findings

Presentation

In uncomplicated complete transposition (i.e. without ventricular septal defect or ductus arteriosus) mixing is dependent upon shunting through a patent foramen ovale. Cyanosis, which is not reversed by administration of 100 per cent oxygen, is the most important single clinical feature. The infants are usually normally developed at birth and central cyanosis persists from this time. Over the first few days of life tachypnoea may supervene. If the condition is not recognized at this stage, increasing cyanosis, metabolic acidosis, and heart failure occur, and the child may die in the first week of life. Apart from cyanosis, physical examination is often normal. Normal splitting of the second heart sound may be difficult to hear. Ejection systolic murmurs may be present.

If there is an associated small ventricular septal defect present, the features will be similar to uncomplicated cases except for an additional pansystolic murmur at the lower left sternal edge.

When the ventricular septal defect is large or there is an associated widely patent ductus, the presenting feature is tachypnoea and there are signs of congestive heart failure. Onset of symptoms will be later than in uncomplicated transposition, typically in the latter part of the first month. Cyanosis may be difficult to detect clinically so that proof of the presence of cyanotic heart disease will require blood gas analysis during administration of 100 per cent oxygen.

Physical examination

Physical examination in patients with complete transposition and a large ventricular septal defect or ductus will reveal increased parasternal and apical cardiac impulses. Co-existent coarctation is not uncommon but in its absence, upper and lower limb pulses will be normal. Splitting of the second heart sound should be audible, possibly with accentuation of the pulmonary component. A pansystolic murmur at the lower left sternal edge accompanies a ventricular septal defect and a continuous murmur just spilling through the second sound may be heard at the upper left sternal border with persistence of a large ductus.

The *chest X-ray* in uncomplicated transposition may be normal. Some degree of cardiomegaly or increased pulmonary vascular markings may be seen but are by no means invariable. The so-called classical 'egg-on-side' appearance of the heart though present only in a minority of cases is of some diagnostic value while absence of the normal neonatal thymic shadow may be striking. The latter, however, is a feature of infants with severe cyanotic heart disease of all types. In the presence of a large ventricular septal defect or ductus, cardiomegaly, and plethora will be expected. The aortic arch is normally left-sided.

In the first week of life the *ECG* in uncomplicated transposition may be normal. Later right ventricular hypertrophy, as evidenced by failure of inversion of T waves in V_4 R and V_1 will usually be seen. The mean frontal QRS axis is typically normal or to the right. With large communications at ventricular or great arterial level, right or biventricular hypertrophy is found, and especially with large ventricular septal

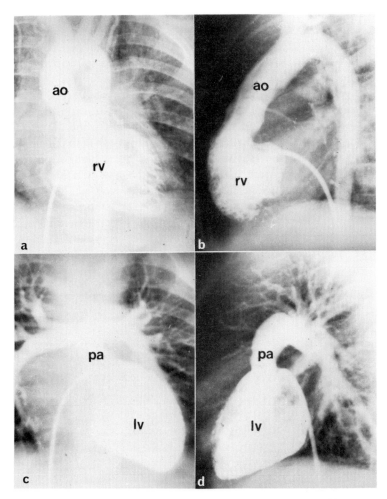

Fig. 27.4 Angiograms from a patient with complete transposition (situs solitus, atrioventricular concordance and ventriculo-arterial discordance). Injection into the right ventricle (rv) in frontal (a) and lateral (b) projections shows an anterior right-sided aorta (ao) arising from the morphologically right ventricle, while injection (c, d) into the morphologically left ventricle (lv) shows a posterior left-sided pulmonary artery (pa) arising from this ventricle.

defects the mean frontal QRS axis may be superior, although the latter is more a feature of univentricular hearts of left ventricular type and transposition (ventriculo-arterial discordance).

Cardiac catheterization should be performed as a matter of urgency in all neonates suspected of having cyanotic congenital heart disease. In no circumstances is this more important than in complete transposition, since in this anomaly not only is the diagnosis confirmed by catheterization, but the initial palliative procedure is undertaken (balloon atrial septostomy). In uncomplicated complete transposition, the catheter passes from the systemic venous ventricle to the aorta. The oxygen saturation in the aorta is considerably lower than in the pulmonary artery. The latter is entered by passing the catheter from right atrium, through the foramen ovale to left atrium, and then through the mitral valve to the left ventricle. This is facilitated by use of the flexible flow guided Swan–Ganz catheter which has a small inflatable balloon at the end. The left ventricular pressure will be lower than in the right ventricle. When a large ventricular septal defect is present, right and left ventricular pressures will be equal and bidirectional shunting

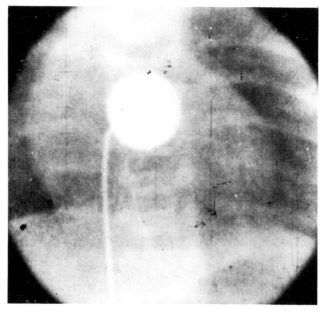

Fig. 27.5 Radiograph of a contrast inflated balloon catheter in the left atrium in a patient with complete transposition prior to atrial septostomy (Rashkind procedure).

occurs at ventricular level. The aortic saturation, however, will still be lower than that in the pulmonary artery.

Angiography should be performed in both ventricles as well as in the aorta, the latter to exclude a ductus and to visualize the anatomy of the aortic arch. Ventricular injections will reveal inappropriate origins of the great arteries (Fig. 27.4).

Treatment

Cardiac catheterization is mandatory as soon as suspicion of transposition is aroused. Once the diagnosis has been confirmed, a Rashkind catheter with an inflatable balloon at its tip is passed through the foramen ovale into the left atrium. It is then inflated with a mixture of radio-opaque contrast material and saline (Fig. 27.5) and then jerked back so as to tear the atrial septum primum. Providing the septum is torn and not merely stretched, this usually facilitates mixing at atrial level. Balloon septostomy should also be carried out in complete transposition plus ventricular septal defect as the ventricular septal defect may close or pulmonary artery banding may be necessary and ventricular mixing hence reduced. If for any reason the atrial septostomy does not achieve an increase in Po_2 to > 30 mmHg some centres would carry out an atrial septectomy (Blalock – Hanlon procedure, see Chapter 11) while others would proceed to Mustard's operation.

At the present time the latter is optimally performed between one year and 18 months. Venous blood is rerouted at atrial level by insertion of an inter-atrial Dacron or pericardial baffle so as to direct the systemic venous return across to the left ventricle and pulmonary artery, while the pulmonary venous return is directed across to the right ventricle and aorta via the tricuspid valve. In uncomplicated transposition Mustard's operation has a mortality even in infancy of under 10 per cent. Long-term results after Mustard's operation are uncertain as it is still a relatively new procedure. Particular complications are development of superior and/or inferior vena caval obstruction, pulmonary venous obstruction, and arrhythmias. Improvements in surgical technique, however, have greatly reduced the frequency of these complications. Senning's operation, which again involves interatrial rerouting of systemic and pulmonary venous returns but utilizes the posterior wall of the aorta as the 'baffle' material may have an equally good if not better long-term prognosis than Mustard's operation.

In the presence of a large ductus or ventricular septal defect the problem is initially of heart failure and subsequently is the risk of developing pulmonary vascular disease. This can be dealt with by early correction or by pulmonary artery banding, corrective surgery being delayed until the child is older. One approach to correction is to close the ventricular septal defect, preferably through the tricuspid valve via a right atrial incision, and then to perform Mustard's operation. Other centres prefer the operation devised by Rastelli where the atrial sep- tum is closed and an interventricular patch is placed so as to form a tunnel from the left ventricle through the ventricular septal defect to aorta. A valved conduit is placed between the right ventricle and pulmonary artery, the latter being excluded from the left ventricle. Either way, the operative mortality is higher than with complete trans- position alone. When a large ductus is present, this requires ligation.

An alternative approach to re-routing blood in transposition is to redirect the circulation at great arterial level. This 'switch' operation involves detaching both great arteries from the ventricles and anas- tomosing them to their appropriate ventricle as well as re-implanting the coronary arteries to the re-sited aorta. This operation, which is experimental at the time of writing, can only be performed if the left ventricular muscle mass is able to sustain systemic pressures. The hospital mortality for transposition plus ventricular septal defect treated by Rastelli's procedure or by Mustard's operation and closure of ventricular septal defect is 5–20 per cent. The anatomic correction switching the great arteries still has a mortality above 50 per cent. In our opinion at present, therefore, use of the switch operation for uncomplicated transposition is totally contraindicated, but there may be a place for this procedure in transposition plus large ventricular septal defect.

COMPLETE TRANSPOSITION WITH PULMONARY STENOSIS

These patients present in a similar manner to those with uncomplicated transposition, but will have an ejection systolic murmur at the upper sternal border. Palliation is carried out by balloon septostomy but corrective surgery poses problems. If pulmonary stenosis is valvar, Mustard's operation and valvotomy are performed but with subvalvar stenosis a direct approach may produce heart block and/or damage the mitral valve apparatus and it may be necessary to place a conduit between left ventricle and pulmonary artery.

COMPLETE TRANSPOSITION WITH VENTRICULAR SEPTAL DEFECT AND PULMONARY STENOSIS

In anatomical terms the heart is identical to complete transposition with ventricular septal defect except for the added factor of pulmonary stenosis, which may be valvar or subvalvar, the latter having several possible anatomical substrates (Fig. 27.3). This combination of anomalies presents in a manner similar to tetralogy of Fallot, although cyanosis is likely to be more severe for a given reduction in pulmonary blood flow. Clinical, ECG, and radiographic findings are also comparable to those of Fallot's tetralogy, although a right aortic arch would not be expected. If cyanosis is severe in the first year of life, a systemic-pulmonary anastomosis should be performed. Corrective surgery depends on the nature of the obstruction to pulmonary blood flow. Uncommonly stenosis is valvar, in which case valvotomy, closure of the ventricular septal defect, and Mustard's operation can be performed. If the stenosis is subvalvar with a good-sized ventricular septal defect, pulmonary venous return to the left atrium can be channelled to the aorta with an intraventricular patch; the pulmonary artery is closed at valve level and a valved conduit placed between the right ventricle and the main pulmonary artery (Rastelli operation). The hospital mortality for this condition is 25 per cent.

References

Anderson, R. H. (1978). Morphogenesis of ventriculo-arterial discordance. In *Embryology and tetralogy of the heart and the great arteries* (ed. L. H. S. Van Mierop, A. Oppenheimer-Dekker, and C. Bruins), pp. 93–111. Boerhaave Series 13. Martinus Nijhoff. The Hague.

Paul, M. H., Van Praagh, S., and Van Praagh, R. (1968) Transposition of the great arteries. In *Paediatric cardiology.* (ed. H. Watson.) Lloyd-Lure, London.

Rashkind, W. J. and Miller, W. W. (1968). Transposition of the great arteries. Results of palliation by balloon atrioseptostomy in thirty-one infants. *Circulation* **38**, 453.

Shaher, R. M. (1973). *Complete transposition of the great arteries.* Academic Press, New York.

Tynan, M. J. (1971). Survival of infants with transposition of great arteries after balloon atrial septostomy. *Lancet* **1**, 621.

28 Corrected transposition

Anatomy and embryology

This form of transposition usually consists of situs solitus, discordant atrioventricular connexions, and discordant ventriculo-arterial connexions but may also exist in situs inversus with the same chamber connexions (Fig. 28.1). The course of the circulation is from right

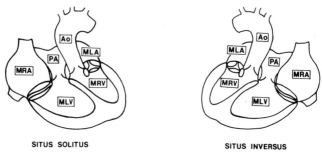

SITUS SOLITUS   SITUS INVERSUS

Fig. 28.1 The chamber combinations to be found in congenitally corrected transposition (atrioventricular discordance *and* ventriculo-arterial discordance). MRA = morphologically right atrium; MLA = morphologically left atrium; MRV = morphologically right ventricle; MLV = morphologically left ventricle; PA = pulmonary artery; AO = aorta.

atrium through mitral valve to the morphologically left ventricle (Fig. 28.2) and thence to a posteriorly situated pulmonary artery. The pulmonary venous return passes from the left atrium through the tricuspid valve to the morphologically right ventricle and is distributed to the body through an anterior, usually left-sided aorta (in situs solitus). When there are no associated anomalies, the patient is asymptomatic and the condition may not be suspected during life; hence the term 'physiologically corrected'. In the majority of cases there are associated anomalies, the most common being ventricular septal defect, pulmonary stenosis, left (tricuspid) atrioventricular valve abnormalities, and conduction disturbances, particularly complete atrioventricular block. The anomaly results from either leftward looping of the ventricular segment of the heart tube occurring in the situs solitus heart, or rightward looping in the situs inversus heart.

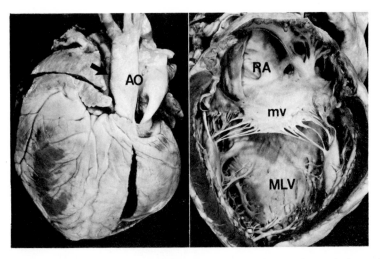

Fig. 28.2 A heart with corrected transposition (situs solitus, atrioventricular and ventriculo-arterial discordance). The aorta (AO) is anterior and to the left of the pulmonary artery (arrowed). It arises from the morphologically right ventricle which is left-sided and receives left atrial blood. The right atrium (RA) drains through a mitral valve (MV) into the morphologically left ventricle (MLV) which gives rise to the pulmonary artery. (Specimen and photographs by courtesy of Dr. A. E. Becker, Amsterdam, the Netherlands.)

Clinical findings

Clinical presentation will depend upon the associated anomalies. When only a ventricular septal defect is present, symptomatology will be as for isolated ventricular septal defect, and will depend on the size of the defect (see Chapter 21). Pulmonary stenosis associated with ventricular septal defect will result in cyanosis, the symptomatology mimicking Fallot's tetralogy. Hypercyanotic attacks, however, will not occur. The condition may present as isolated heart block, frequently developing in adolescence. Rarely left (tricuspid) atrioventricular valve incompetence (left-sided Ebstein's anomaly) may be severe with clinical features mimicking 'mitral incompetence' (Fig. 28.3b).

Physical examination may suggest the diagnosis of corrected transposition by the finding of a particularly loud and often palpable aortic component to the second heart sound in the second or third left intercostal space. *Chest X-ray* characteristically reveals a straight upper left heart border due to the left-sided ascending aorta. Alternatively, dextrocardia may be present with situs solitus. When corrected

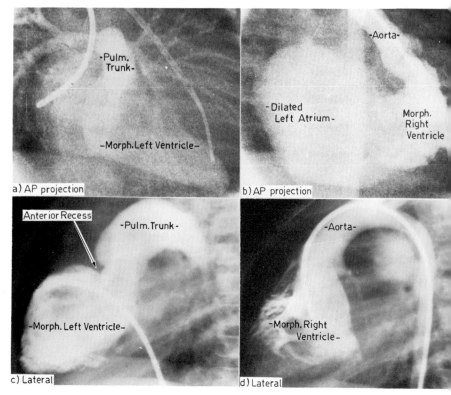

Fig. 28.3 Angiograms performed in frontal view in a patient with physiologically corrected transposition (situs solitus, discordant atrioventricular and discordant ventriculo-arterial connexions). In (a) contrast has been injected into the morphologically right atrium which then passes across the mitral valve into the morphologically left ventricle supporting the pulmonary artery. In (b) retrograde arterial catheterization allows injection into the morphologically right ventricle demonstrating severe left (tricuspid) atrioventricular valve incompetence. Gross dilatation of the left atrium is demonstrated and the anomaly represents the left-sided Ebstein's lesion. (c) and (d) represent morphologically left and right ventricular injections respectively taken in the lateral projection from a different patient. In (c) the posteriorly placed pulmonary artery is seen to arise from the morphologically left ventricle and the characteristic anterior recess is demonstrated. In (d) the heavily trabeculated morphologically right ventricle gives rise to ascending aorta.

transposition exists with situs inversus the identification of isolated laevocardia may suggest the anomaly.

The characteristic *ECG* features (Fig. 7.4) of corrected transposition with situs solitus are the presence of deep right-sided Q-waves (V_4R and V_1) and the absence of the normal left-sided Q-waves in V_6

and V_7. In addition, first-degree block or complete heart block may be present.

At *cardiac catheterization* it may be difficult to pass the catheter from the ventricle receiving systemic venous return to the pulmonary artery, although the aorta may be entered through a ventricular septal defect (if present) and found to be left-sided. The diagnosis is confirmed by angiography, which reveals atrioventricular discordance (Fig. 28.3). Pressures and oxymetry are dependent upon associated anomalies.

Treatment

Management is also dependent upon the associated anomalies. In patients with a ventricular septal defect and pulmonary outflow obstruction when pulmonary blood flow is limited, in early life palliation by means of a systemic artery/pulmonary artery anastomosis is appropriate. If there is excessive pulmonary flow (ventricular septal defect with no pulmonary stenosis), then banding of the main pulmonary artery can be carried out. Large ventricular septal defects are closed surgically through the morphologically left ventricle or the mitral valve, but it is vitally important for the surgeon to appreciate the unusual anterior situation of the atrioventricular conduction tissue

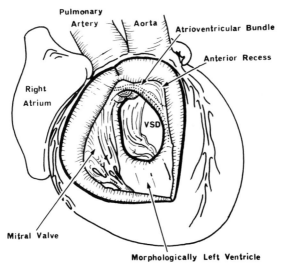

Fig. 28.4 Artist's impression showing the course of the atrioventricular conduction tissue (illustrated by the dotted lines) which passes in front of the pulmonary outflow tract and above the ventricular septal defect. Reproduced with permission from Anderson and Shinebourne: *Paediatric Cardiology, 1977*, Churchill Livingstone, Edinburgh.

(Fig. 28.4). This necessitates closure of the ventricular septal defect by placing the sutures for the patch closure on the left side of the ventricular septal defect, in contra-distinction to the usual type of ventricular septal defect. The proximity of the bundle to the pulmonary outflow tract also influences relief of pulmonary stenosis. Direct relief of subvalvar muscular stenosis is absolutely contraindicated since such resection will remove the atrioventricular bundle and cause heart block. Relief of right ventricular outflow tract obstruction is carried out by means of an external tube conduit, leaving the existing pulmonary outflow tract in continuity.

References

Allwork, S. P., Bentall, H. H., Becker, A. E., Cameron, H., Gerlis, L. M., Wilkinson, J. L., and Anderson, R. H. (1976). Congenitally corrected transposition of the great arteries: Morphologic study of 32 cases. *American Journal of Cardiology* **38**, 910.

Anderson, R. H., Becker, A. E., Arnold, R., and Wilkinson, J. L. (1974). The conducting tissues in congenitally corrected transposition. *Circulation* **50**, 911.

Friedberg, D. Z. and Nadas, A. S. (1970). Clinical profile of patients with congenitally corrected transposition of the great arteries: a study of 60 cases. *New England Journal of Medicine* **282**, 1053.

Losekoot, T. G. (1978). Conditions with atrioventricular discordance—clinical investigation. In *Paediatric cardiology, 1977* (ed. R. H. Anderson and E. A. Shinebourne), pp. 198–206. Churchill Livingstone, Edinburgh.

Soto, B., Bargeron, L. M., Bream, P. R., and Elliott, L. P. (1978). Conditions with atrioventricular discordance—angiographic study. In *Paediatric cardiology, 1977* (ed. R. H. Anderson and E. A. Shinebourne), pp. 207–21. Churchill Livingstone, Edinburgh.

29 Double outlet ventricles

Definitions

The term 'double outlet ventricle' defines an abnormal ventriculo-arterial connexion where more than half of each great artery arises from the same ventricle, be it right or left. For completeness, atrial situs and atrioventricular connexion must also be stated. Thus double outlet arterial connexion can be found with situs solitus, inversus or ambiguus, and with any form of atrioventricular connexion. As well as taking origin from right or left ventricle, both arteries can arise from an outlet chamber or the main chamber of a univentricular heart. In view of the rarity of the other varieties of double outlet ventricles, most attention will be confined to double outlet right ventricle (DORV) in situs solitus with atrioventricular concordance.

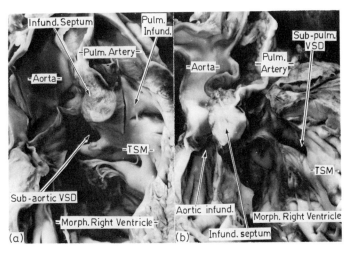

Fig. 29.1 The position of the ventricular septal defect in double outlet right ventricle with concordant atrioventricular connexions and sub-aortic defect (a) and sub-pulmonary defect (b). The latter anomaly is frequently termed the Taussig–Bing malformation.

DOUBLE OUTLET RIGHT VENTRICLE WITH CONCORDANT ATRIOVENTRICULAR CONNEXIONS

Anatomy and embryology

A ventricular septal defect is almost invariable and is either subaortic (Fig. 29.1a) or subpulmonary (Fig. 29.1b). When the defect is subpulmonary, the malformation is frequently termed the Taussig–Bing anomaly. Rarely the ventricular septal defect may be beneath both great arteries (doubly committed) or neither (uncommitted). The aorta in double outlet right ventricle is usually to the right of the pulmonary artery but may be left-sided. It is usual to find a muscular infundibulum beneath both arterial valves (bilateral infundibula) so that there is discontinuity between the arterial and atrioventricular valves. However, presence of atrioventricular arterial valve continuity does not exclude the diagnosis of double outlet ventricle. In terms of anatomy, hearts with double outlet right ventricle reflect their embryological origin. Thus, during development the aorta initially arises above the developing right ventricle and is transferred to the left ventricle (see Chapter 13). Hearts exist which reflect arrested development of this process, and so a spectrum is found between double outlet right ventricle with sub-aortic defect and isolated ventricular septal defect with overriding aorta. Whether or not there is arterial-atrioventricular valvar continuity depends on whether or not the inner heart curvature is reabsorbed during development. It is for this reason that we use the '50 per cent rule' to determine if a heart has a double outlet connexion or arterial concordance. A similar series of anomalies is seen when the ventricular septal defect is in sub-pulmonary position, but this time the series extends between double outlet and complete transposition (arterial discordance). Again the series is divided at the 50 per cent point, irrespective of the morphology of the outflow tract.

Associated anomalies are frequent with double outlet right ventricle, particularly arterial stenosis. Pulmonary stenosis is seen most frequently when the defect is sub-aortic, and is usually infundibular in origin although valvar stenosis may be found. Aortic infundibular stenosis is a frequent finding when the defect is sub-pulmonary, as are the usual accompaniments of reduced aortic flow, namely, coarctation and isthmal hypoplasia. Straddling mitral valve is also frequently found with double outlet right ventricle and sub-pulmonary defect.

The particular form of double outlet right ventricle in which a bilateral infundibulum is found is rare. Using the definition of double outlet ventricle presently employed, however, this abnormal ventriculo-arterial connexion will be encountered more frequently since many hearts with the morphology of tetralogy of Fallot have the ventriculo-arterial connexion of double outlet right ventricle (as well as a subaortic ventricular septal defect) while some hearts loosely termed 'transposition of the great arteries and VSD' have double outlet right ventricle with subpulmonary ventricular septal defect.

Clinical findings

Presentation
This depends on the position of the ventricular septal defect, the magnitude of pulmonary blood flow, and the presence or absence of additional anomalies, in particular coarctation of the aorta. When the defect is subaortic, the highly oxygenated pulmonary venous return streams from the left ventricle to the aorta (Fig. 29.2b). As with tetralogy of Fallot, the degree of arterial desaturation or cyanosis is then dependent on pulmonary stenosis. When the defect is subpulmonary (Taussig–Bing anomaly), the haemodynamic disturbance mimics that of complete transposition with ventricular septal defect as the pulmonary venous return streams back to the pulmonary artery (Fig.

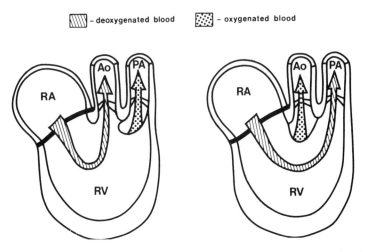

Fig. 29.2 Diagrammatic representation of the flow pattern in double outlet right ventricle with sub-pulmonary defect (left-hand diagram). The pulmonary venous return streams preferentially through the ventricular septal defect into the pulmonary artery while systemic venous return passes predominantly to aorta. On the right-hand diagram the flow patterns are shown in a sub-aortic defect where pulmonary venous return streams preferentially through the ventricular septal defect to the aorta.

29.2a). Coarctation of the aorta is common with subpulmonary defects and tends to exacerbate heart failure.

Subaortic defects without pulmonary stenosis have clinical findings similar to large ventricular septal defects but minimal arterial desaturation is present. When pulmonary stenosis is present, the findings are as in tetralogy of Fallot (Chapter 23). Subpulmonary defects are similar to complete transposition with ventricular septal defect (Chapter 27).

Physical examination
Chest X-ray is non-specific. Pulmonary vascular markings will be

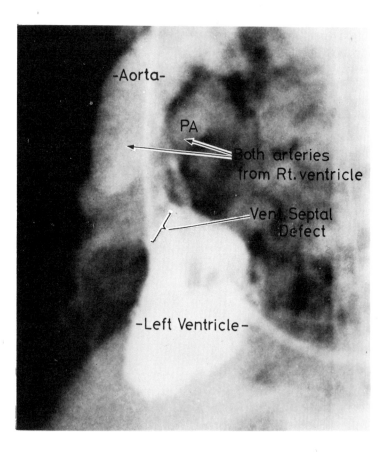

Fig. 29.3 Lateral view of left ventricular angiogram in a patient with double outlet right ventricle and subaortic VSD.

increased in the absence and reduced in the presence of severe pulmonary stenosis, but will be normal with moderate pulmonary stenosis. A straight upper left heart border may suggest double outlet right ventricle with left-sided aorta. The *ECG* will show right ventricular hypertrophy but is also non-specific. Some defects exhibit a superior axis which may help in differential diagnosis from tetralogy of Fallot or alert to the possibility of more complex anatomy. When two great arteries are demonstrated using *echocardiography*, their relationship to the ventricular septum can be diagnostic. At *cardiac catheterization* equal right and left ventricular pressures are the rule but occasionally a closing ventricular septal defect results in higher left ventricular systolic pressures. With subaortic defects there is a left-to-right shunt at ventricular level. Some degree of arterial desaturation will be found but the saturation in the aorta will be higher than in the pulmonary artery. When the ventricular septal defect is subpulmonary the findings will be as in complete transposition with ventricular septal defect: bidirectional shunting at ventricular level is usual but with the saturation in aorta being lower than in the pulmonary artery. A left ventriculogram as well as a right is mandatory (Fig. 29.3). An aortogram is required for exclusion of a persistent ductus arteriosus or coarctation. The chosen projection for ventriculography should profile the ventricular septum so as to clarify the ventriculo-arterial connexion.

Treatment
In double outlet right ventricle with subpulmonary ventricular septal defect (Taussig–Bing anomaly) a balloon septostomy should be carried out at cardiac catheterization. Patients with double outlet ventricle may be symptomatic early in life because of increased or decreased pulmonary blood flow (associated pulmonary stenosis). In the latter a systemic artery/pulmonary artery anastomosis, and in the former banding of the main pulmonary artery can be carried out as palliative procedures. Total correction is then performed at a later date, usually around the age of five or six years.

The concept of corrective surgery is based upon re-routing blood from the left ventricle into the aorta, by means of an interventricular baffle. This can be readily performed in patients with a ventricular septal defect in the subaortic position. Subsequent relief of pulmonary stenosis when present, can be carried out using a plastic repair or an external tube conduit. When the ventricular septal defect is in the subpulmonary position, it is not possible to place an interventricular baffle to re-route blood from left ventricle into the aorta without causing obstruction to pulmonary flow. Therefore in this anomaly the interventricular patch is placed so as to include the pulmonary valve with the left ventricle, following which Mustard's operation (see Chapter 27) is performed to redirect systemic and pulmonary venous returns at atrial level.

Total correction of either form of double outlet right ventricle (with atrioventricular concordance) carries a mortality of 5–20 per cent.

DOUBLE OUTLET RIGHT VENTRICLE WITH ATRIOVENTRICULAR DISCORDANCE

This rare anomaly has similar atrial and ventricular anatomy to congenitally corrected transposition plus ventricular septal defect (atrial situs solitus or inversus with discordant atrioventricular and discordant ventriculo-arterial connexions plus ventricular septal defect). In double outlet right ventricle with atrioventricular discordance the right atrium connects (via the mitral valve) with the left

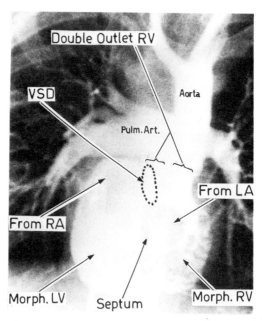

Fig. 29.4 Injection into the morphologically left ventricle in a patient with situs solitus, discordant atrioventricular connexions, and double outlet right ventricle. Contrast passes from the smooth walled left ventricle across the ventricular septal defect and into the trabeculated morphologically right ventricle. The ventricular septal defect is sub-pulmonary and the aorta left sided.

ventricle, sole egress from which is a ventricular septal defect (Fig. 29.4). Both great arteries arise from the morphologically right ventricle, the ventricular septal defect characteristically being subpulmonary. Subvalvar pulmonary stenosis is also commonly associated.

Clinical presentation, ECG, and chest X-ray are identical to those of corrected transposition with ventricular septal defect ± pulmonary stenosis as are the findings at cardiac catheterization. Definitive correction involves closure of the ventricular septal defect (avoiding the abnormally placed conduction tissue) and placing a conduit from (morphologically) left ventricle to pulmonary artery.

DOUBLE OUTLET LEFT VENTRICLE
Although in the past this anomaly had been thought not to be embryologically possible—always a dangerous statement!—many examples have now been described. None-the-less, it remains exceedingly rare. As would be expected it has been described with situs solitus or inversus, with concordant or discordant atrioventricular connexions, and with subpulmonary or subaortic ventricular septal defects. Pulmonary stenosis, coarctation, or other anomalies may be associated and these dominate the clinical picture. Further discussion of such a rare anomaly is not warranted in this book.

DOUBLE OUTLET OUTLET CHAMBER OR MAIN CHAMBER OF UNIVENTRICULAR HEART
This type of abnormal ventriculo-arterial connexion in univentricular hearts is usually the least of the patient's problems. As the rest of the cardiac anatomy is more important in determining clinical features and the possibilities for surgical treatment, double outlet outlet chamber and double outlet main chamber of univentricular heart will not be considered further in this section.

References

Anderson, R. H., Wilkinson, J. L., Arnold, R., Becker, A. E., and Lubkiewicz, K. (1974). Morphogenesis of bulboventricular malformations. II. Observations on malformed hearts. *British Heart Journal* **36**, 948.

Brandt, P. W. T., Calder, A. L., Barratt-Boyes, B. G., and Neutze, J. M. (1976). Double outlet left ventricle. Morphology, cineangiographic diagnosis and surgical treatment. *American Journal of Cardiology* **38**, 897.

Hallerman, F. J., Kincaid, O. W., Ritter, D. G., Ongley, P. A., and Titus, J. L. (1970). Angiographic and anatomic findings in origin of both great arteries from the right ventricle. *American Journal of Roentgenology* **109**, 51.

Lev, M., Bharati, S., Meng, C. C. L., Liberthson, R. R., Paul, M. H., and Idriss, F. (1972). A concept of double outlet right ventricle. *Journal of Thoracic and Cardiovascular Surgery* **64**, 271.

Lincoln, C., Anderson, R. H., Shinebourne, E. A., English, T. A. H., and Wilkinson, J. L. (1975). Double outlet right ventricle with l-malposition of the aorta. *British Heart Journal* **36**, 948.

30 Truncus arteriosus

Anatomy and embryology

Truncus arteriosus is defined as a single trunk exiting from the heart through a single arterial valve and giving rise to ascending aorta, pulmonary arteries, and coronary arteries. It results from failure of septation of the embryonic truncus by the infundibular truncal ridges. It can be subdivided depending on the precise origin of the pulmonary arteries, the principle types being a single main pulmonary artery (Type I) (Fig. 30.1a), or separate right and left pulmonary arteries (Type II and III) (Fig. 30.1b). The term truncus Type IV has been applied to some examples of the anomaly of pulmonary atresia with ventricular septal defect, but the 'single' arterial trunk in this instance

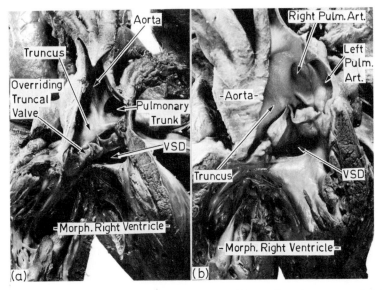

Fig. 30.1 The morphology of truncus arteriosus with a main pulmonary trunk (a) and a truncus arteriosus with separate origin of the right and left pulmonary arteries from the ascending trunk (b). The former anomaly is the Type I of Collet and Edwards while the latter anomaly and its related partner in which the right and left pulmonary arteries arise from the side of the truncus are Types II and III respectively.

is usually an aorta. The truncus usually straddles the ventricular septum and there is, perforce, a high ventricular septal defect. The truncal valve has between two and six cusps.

Incidence
This anomaly is uncommon.

Clinical findings
Heart failure, often occurring towards the end of the first month, is the presenting feature. Since truncus arteriosus produces a common mixing situation, there will be arterial desaturation, but this is often difficult to detect clinically. However, it will be easily identified by blood gas analysis after administration of 100 per cent oxygen. Biventricular hypertrophy and bounding pulses are often present. On auscultation the second sound should be single, and an ejection click will be heard as well as a systolic murmur. When truncal valve incompetence occurs, a diastolic murmur will be present.

Chest X-ray shows cardiomegaly and plethora. A main pulmonary artery is not seen, and the right and left pulmonary arteries may exhibit

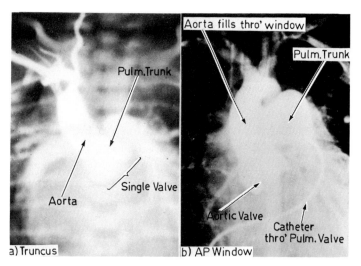

Fig. 30.2 Angiograms illustrating the difference between truncus arteriosus and aorto-pulmonary window. (a) shows a truncus arteriosus. The arterial valve supports both the aorta and the pulmonary trunk. (b) shows an aorto-pulmonary window in the frontal projection. Catheter has passed through the pulmonary valve into the main pulmonary artery where injection has been made. Contrast then passes across to outline the aorta and aortic valve.

a high 'take-off'. A right aortic arch may be found. The *ECG* exhibits a variable QRS axis and right, left, or biventricular hypertrophy. *Cardiac catheterization* will demonstrate equal ventricular pressures with bidirectional shunting at ventricular or great artery level, and arterial desaturation. Angiography should be performed in both ventricles and in the arterial trunk arising from the heart. Care must be taken to distinguish truncus arteriosus (Fig. 30.2a) from aorto-pulmonary window (Fig. 30.2b, see Chapter 31) on the angiogram.

Treatment
Heart failure is treated medically. If unsuccessful, surgical intervention is required. In infancy, pulmonary artery banding, bilateral if necessary, may be performed and total correction carried out when the child is about five years old. In truncus arteriosus, the corrective procedure (Rastelli) is to close the ventricular septal defect so that the left ventricle drains to the common trunk. The pulmonary artery is detached from the back of the trunk and connected to the right ventricle using a tubular valved conduit. Such a regimen of initial palliation and subsequent correction has a considerable mortality and some centres would now advocate total correction as an initial procedure in infancy. The hospital mortality for this condition is 20–30 per cent.

References

Collett, R. W. and Edwards, J. E. (1949). Persistent truncus arteriosus: A classification according to anatomic types. *Surgical Clinics of North America* **29**, 1245.

Crupi, G. C., Macartney, F. J., and Anderson, R. H. (1977). Persistent truncus arteriosus: a study of 66 autopsy cases with special reference to definition and morphogenesis. *American Journal of Cardiology* **40**, 569.

McGoon, D. C., Rastelli, G. C., and Ongley, P. A. (1968). An operation for the correction of truncus arteriosus. *Journal of the American Medical Association* **205**, 69.

Tandon, R., Hauck, A. J., and Nadas, A. S. (1963). Persistent truncus arteriosus: A clinical, haemodynamic and autopsy study of 19 cases. *Circulation* **28**, 1050.

31 Aorto-pulmonary window

Anatomy and embryogenesis
The defect consists of an abnormal communication between ascending aorta and main pulmonary trunk (Fig. 31.1). It represents incomplete development and fusion of the extra-cardiac aortico-pulmonary septum with the truncus septum.

Clinical findings
This rare anomaly is important to recognize as it can be easily repaired

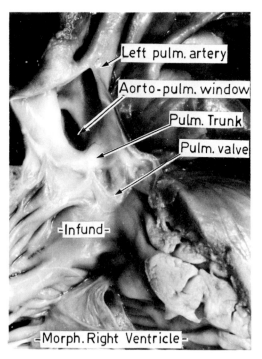

Fig. 31.1 The pulmonary artery of a patient with aorto-pulmonary window. Note the communication between the pulmonary trunk and the ascending part of the aorta. There is additionally interruption of the aortic arch.

on cardiopulmonary bypass. Small defects have similar features to a persistent ductus arteriosus with a continuous murmur and increased pulses. Most defects, however, are large enough to equalize pressures in aorta and pulmonary artery. Under these circumstances, a harsh systolic murmur is heard and differential diagnosis is primarily from a ventricular septal defect. When pulmonary vascular disease develops, there are no murmurs, a loud pulmonary component to the second sound being the striking auscultatory features.

The *chest X-ray* shows cardiomegaly and plethora, although if pulmonary vascular resistance fails to fall post-natally, the lung fields may be normal. The *ECG* shows biventricular hypertrophy. At *cardiac catheterization* the catheter characteristically passes from pulmonary artery to ascending aorta and thence to the head and neck arteries. A step-up in oxygen saturation, together with an elevated pressure, are found in the pulmonary artery. Angiography distinguishes the anomaly from truncus arteriosus (Fig. 30.2).

Treatment

Palliation is not carried out. Surgical closure on cardiopulmonary bypass is best achieved via the aorta. The defect can then be patched from inside the aorta avoiding the coronary ostia. Since there is a primary defect in the aortopulmonary septum, it is necessary to close it by means of a Dacron prosthesis. It is not appropriate to close the defect by direct suture, since this would cause distortion of the great vessels. The hospital mortality for correction of this anomaly is 0–5 per cent.

Reference

Deverall, P. B., Lincoln, J. C. R., Aberdeen, E., Bonham-Carter, R. E., and Waterston, D. J. (1969). Aortopulmonary window. *Journal of Thoracic and Cardiovascular Surgery* **57**, 479.

32 Persistent ductus arteriosus

Anatomy, embryology, and physiology

The ductus arteriosus is that portion of the sixth aortic arch present in the normal fetus which connects the junction of the main and left pulmonary arteries to the descending aorta (Fig. 32.1). Postnatal ductal closure normally occurs in the first week of life in infants born at full term. Closure may be delayed in premature infants, this is thought to be related to higher levels of circulating prostaglandins (E series). Initial constriction of the ductus occurs in response to the increase in oxygen tension accompanying the change from intra- to extrauterine life. Constriction commences at the pulmonary insertion of the ductus. Anatomical closure is dependent upon cicatrization and fibrosis of the constricted ductus. This occurs within the first year of life, converting the ductus to the ligamentum arteriosum.

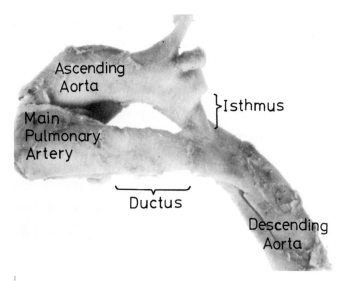

Fig. 32.1 Photograph illustrating the normal ductus arteriosus of a newborn.

Incidence

Persistence of the ductus arteriosus is one of the commonest congenital cardiovascular anomalies. The incidence increases dramatically in populations living at altitude, being 30 times greater at 5000 m than at sea-level. This reflects the lower oxygen tensions at these heights. Rubella virus has been isolated from the ductus arteriosus in infants whose mothers contracted this infection in the first trimester of pregnancy, thus accounting for the high frequency of persistent ductus in 'rubella babies'.

A persistent ductus arteriosus can be found in association with virtually all other intracardiac anomalies and this is dealt with elsewhere in the book.

Clinical findings

Presentation

This is dependent upon the size of the ductus and the level of the pulmonary vascular resistance. Most frequently the ductus is partially constricted. In such circumstances the child will be asymptomatic, and presentation depends on detection of a continuous murmur at auscultation. Thus many patients are diagnosed at the infant welfare clinic or at initial school examination. When the ductus is large, infants born at term present with heart failure, usually in the second month of life. Development of the left-to-right shunt is also dependent on post-natal fall in pulmonary vascular resistance. Premature babies, in whom pulmonary vascular resistance falls rapidly after birth, typically manifest signs of overt cardiac failure in the first week of life. Alternatively, some infants present with failure to thrive in the first few months of life and have recurrent respiratory infections. Rarely when the pulmonary vascular resistance is grossly elevated, there may be right-to-left shunting with cyanosis confined to the lower body. Clubbing would then be more marked in toes than fingers.

Physical examination

When the ductus is small the child will be normally developed and well. Abnormal physical findings are likely to be restricted to auscultation. The heart sounds will be normal but a continuous murmur will be audible, maximal in the second left intercostal space at the left sternal edge. By 'continuous' is meant that the murmur commences in systole and extends through the second heart sound into diastole. The murmur does not have to be heard throughout the entire cardiac cycle. When this is the case, the term 'machinery murmur' is used. The *chest X-ray* may well be normal, although slight increase in pulmonary vascular markings may be observed. The *ECG* also will be normal, although voltage criteria for early left ventricular hypertrophy may be present.

When the ductus is large, there may be signs of heart failure with tachypnoea and hepatomegaly. Pulses in all limbs are bounding, reflecting an increased pulse pressure. This is the consequence of a large left ventricular stroke volume, together with a rapid fall in pressure as blood shunts ('run-off') to the low resistance pulmonary circuit. Parasternal and apical impulses are prominent. The first heart sound is normal and the second closely split. A loud continuous murmur will be heard, possibly accompanied by an apical diastolic murmur as a consequence of increased flow across the mitral valve.

If the pulmonary vascular resistance is raised, the pulmonary component of the second sound becomes louder. At the same time, the continuous murmur becomes shorter so that it only just extends into diastole. A situation may be reached in which the pulmonary and systemic resistances are equal. At such times, either no murmur will be present or only a soft systolic murmur will be audible. This situation may be encountered either in the Eisenmenger syndrome or, more commonly, in the infant prior to post-natal fall in pulmonary vascular resistance.

In the presence of a large ductus, the *chest X-ray* shows cardiomegaly and pulmonary plethora. A left aortic arch is normally present and there is left atrial enlargement. The *ECG* shows sinus rhythm and normal P-waves and P–R interval. Evidence of left ventricular hypertrophy is present, without left-sided T-wave changes. In the first few weeks of life, or in the presence of increased pulmonary vascular resistance, evidence of biventricular hypertrophy will be found.

At *cardiac catheterization* a small step-up in oxygen saturation is found at pulmonary artery level when the communication is small. Pressures will be essentially normal, with occasional minimal elevation of right ventricular and pulmonary artery pressures. When the ductus is large, systolic pressures in aorta and pulmonary artery, and hence in the ventricles, will be equal. Oxygen saturations will reveal a left-to-right shunt at the level of the pulmonary artery. As pulmonary vascular resistance increases, so the magnitude of the shunt decreases until eventually the shunt is reversed. In the latter circumstance, descending aortic oxygen saturation is lower than that in the ascending aorta. During catheterization in patients with large defects, the catheter usually passes easily from the pulmonary artery to the descending aorta. Should this not occur, then a possible diagnosis of aorto-pulmonary window should be considered. Angiography may not be necessary, but an aortogram demarcates the anatomy (Fig. 4.1) and distinguishes a ductus from an aorto-pulmonary window, ventricular septal defect with aortic incompetence, or other causes of a continuous murmur (Chapter 35).

Treatment

The diagnosis is usually apparent on clinical examination, and if so cardiac catheterization may be unnecessary although in our opinion preferable. It is imperative in these circumstances to perform blood gas sampling in 100 per cent oxygen to rule out cyanotic heart disease (see p. 23). Surgical closure by ligation, transection, or direct suture is indicated in all older children and in symptomatic infants. Heart failure in infancy should be treated with digoxin, diuretics, and potassium supplements. Heart failure in premature infants should be treated similarly, and in some the ductus will close spontaneously. Recently, prostaglandin synthetase inhibitors such as indomethacin or aspirin have been used to encourage ductal closure in this group, but with variable success. The reasons for closure in asymptomatic patients are first to prevent development of possible pulmonary vascular disease, and secondly to diminish the risk of subacute bacterial endocarditis. Should the latter develop and be resistant to bactericidal therapy, surgical excision of the infected ductus may be performed. Should the Eisenmenger syndrome supervene, surgical closure is contra-indicated. The hospital mortality for this condition should be 0 per cent.

References

Cassels, D. E. (1973). *The ductus arteriosus.* Charles C. Thomas. Springfield, Ill.

Heymann, M. A., Rudolph, A. M., and Silverman, N. H. (1976). Closure of the ductus arterious in premature infants by inhibition of prostaglandin synthesis. *New England Journal of Medicine* **295**, 530.

Rowe, R. D. (1978). Patent ductus arteriosus. In *Heart disease in infancy and childhood* (ed. Keith, J. D., Rowe, R. D., and Vlad, P.), Chapter 24. Macmillan, New York.

Rudolph, A. M. (1978). The ductus arteriosus. In *Paediatric cardiology, 1977* (ed. Anderson, R. H. and Shinebourne, E. A.), Chapter 47. Churchill Livingstone, Edinburgh.

33 Pulmonary stenosis

Anatomy and embryology

Isolated pulmonary stenosis occurs at the level of the pulmonary valve or rarely at infundibular level. An anomalous muscle bundle of the right ventricle can produce similar clinical features, although the latter is usually associated with a ventricular septal defect. Valvar stenosis is usually of the 'domed' variety with a central orifice and fused commissures although a slit-like bicuspid orifice can occur. Severe or critical stenosis in infancy merges imperceptibly into the anomaly of pulmonary atresia with intact septum, although the right ventricle is usually larger in the former. There is hypertrophy of the right ventricular myocardium. Valvar pulmonary stenosis results from fusion of the pulmonary valve cusps during middle to late intra-uterine development. Supravalvar pulmonary stenosis is exceptionally rare, but may accompany hypercalcaemia in infancy. Peripheral pulmonary stenosis may occur as a consequence of rubella or administration of drugs such as thalidomide.

Incidence

Mild to moderate pulmonary stenosis is a common cardiac defect in children and adults. Critical pulmonary stenosis as a cause of profound cyanosis in the neonatal period is not uncommon in a paediatric cardiology referral centre.

Clinical findings

Critical pulmonary stenosis presents in the neonatal period in a fashion similar to pulmonary atresia with intact septum (see Chapter 24). The paucity of right-sided forces on the *ECG*, however, may be less marked. Distinction between the two is made by right ventricular angiography following catheterization, when a pin-hole meatus will be seen in the stenosed pulmonary valve.

Pulmonary stenosis presents more frequently in older children with a systolic murmur, usually detected at routine examination. Patients are asymptomatic. In contrast to neonates with critical stenosis, cyanosis is only present if there is an additional atrial septal defect (or patent foramen ovale). If the stenosis is severe in the older child, there may be effort dyspnoea and very rarely heart failure or angina on effort may supervene.

On examination a prominent parasternal impulse reflects right ventricular hypertrophy. The pulmonary component of the second sound will be soft and delayed, the extent of delay depending on the severity of stenosis. In severe stenosis, the second heart sound is single (aortic closure). An ejection systolic murmur is present, maximal in the second or third left intercostal space. The murmur peaks in early to mid-systole but, with increasing stenosis, peaks later. An ejection click accompanies non-severe valvar stenosis. It is usually heard maximally at the upper left sternal edge. *Chest X-ray* shows marked post-stenotic dilatation of the pulmonary artery (Fig. 7.3 cf. tetralogy of Fallot; Fig. 7.1a). The peripheral pulmonary vascular markings are normal in the absence of an intra-atrial communication, rather than reduced as is commonly assumed. Heart size is normal unless stenosis is severe and there is heart failure. The *ECG* exhibits right ventricular

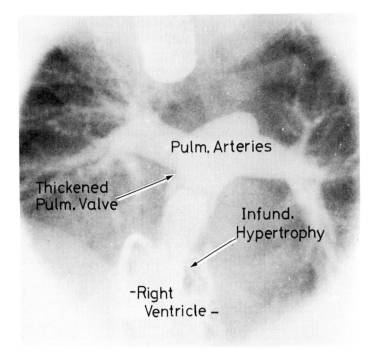

Fig. 33.1 Right ventriculogram in patient with severe valvar pulmonary stenosis. The thickened domed valve is shown and there is secondary infundibular hypertrophy.

hypertrophy, the height of the R-waves in V_4R and V_1 giving a good indication of the degree of hypertrophy and hence the severity of stenosis. With severe stenosis, there may be T-wave inversion across the chest leads to V_6. With gross hypertrophy, the right ventricle enlarges to form the cardiac apex and V_5 and V_6 reflect right ventricular strain. *Cardiac catheterization* will reveal increased right ventricular but normal to low pulmonary artery pressures. Right ventriculography is mandatory in order to demarcate precise anatomy (Fig. 33.1). This will also indicate any additional and perhaps unsuspected anomalies.

Treatment

If stenosis is mild and right ventricular pressure is less than 60 mmHg, no treatment is indicated. In general, more severe stenosis with higher pressures will require surgical relief of the obstruction, and it is unwise to wait until gross right ventricular hypertrophy has developed. Pulmonary valvotomy alone is employed for valvar stenosis even when there is moderate secondary infundibular stenosis. With severe infundibular stenosis there is a place for resection of infundibular muscle and if the pulmonary valve ring is very small a transannular patch may be required.

References

Lucas, R. V. and Moller, H. J. (1970). Pulmonary valvular stenosis. *Cardiovascular Clinics* **2**, 155.

Rowe, R. D. (1978). Pulmonary stenosis with normal aortic root. In *Heart disease in infancy and childhood* (ed. Keith, J. D., Rowe, R. D., and Vlad, P.). Macmillan, New York.

34 Congenital aortic stenosis and incompetence

AORTIC STENOSIS

Anatomy
Aortic stenosis is usually valvar but may be subvalvar or supravalvar, *Valvar stenosis* is most frequently associated with a bicuspid valve although infants dying from severe aortic stenosis may have a thickened mucocartilagenous domed 'unicuspid' valve. *Subvalvar* stenosis is usually caused by a fibromuscular diaphragm of tissue which forms a constrictive ring round the septum and the facing surface of the antero-septal leaflet of the mitral valve. In some cases the diaphragm may be elongated to form a stenotic tunnel. Subvalvar stenosis due to hypertrophic obstructive cardiomyopathy is considered elsewhere (Chapter 41). Some patients with supravalvar aortic stenosis have in addition mental retardation, a characteristic 'elfin' facies, other arterial stenoses, particularly pulmonary, and unexplained hypercalcaemia in infancy. Experimental work supports an association between a disorder of calcium metabolism in the fetus and some cases of supravalvar aortic stenosis. When large doses of Vitamin D were fed to pregnant animals, this induced hypercalcaemia in the fetus and subsequent aortic abnormalities in the offspring similar to those of supravalvar stenosis in man. The coronary arteries in supravalvar stenosis, which are perfused at high pressure as their ostia are proximal to the obstruction, may be thick walled, dilated, and tortuous.

Incidence
A bicuspid aortic valve is one of the commonest congenital cardiac anomalies. However, it frequently does not produce symptoms until later life. Thus calcific aortic stenosis in middle age is often a result of this congenital anomaly. When isolated, it is rare for aortic stenosis to be a consequence of rheumatic heart disease. Severe aortic stenosis in infancy is a rare cause of heart failure in the first week of life and whenever present associated coarctation must always be excluded, since reduced aortic flow will predispose to isthmal hypoplasia.

Clinical findings

Mild to moderately severe stenosis does not give rise to symptoms. Clinical presentation is by a systolic murmur detected at incidental examination. When severe, usually in older patients, aortic stenosis can give rise to effort dyspnoea, syncope on exercise, or angina of effort. Presentation of severe stenosis in infancy is with heart failure, and if severe, may mimic the hypoplastic left heart syndrome. In mild valvar aortic stenosis, examination will reveal an ejection systolic murmur maximal in the second right intercostal space. An aortic ejection click is usually present, heard most easily at the apex. If more severe the pulse volume will be reduced and a slow rising (anacrotic) pulse will be palpated. A prominent heaving apical pulsation indicates left ventricular hypertrophy, and a thrill is often palpable in the second right intercostal space (aortic area). The second heart sound may appear single and eventually reversed splitting will be audible, with delay in the second (aortic) component being more apparent in expiration. Many cases of congenital aortic stenosis also exhibit mild aortic incompetence and an early diastolic murmur will therefore be audible at the left sternal edge in the third space. A fourth heart sound may be audible. In supravalvar or subvalvar stenosis it is rare to hear an ejection click. Characteristically in supravalvar stenosis the pulse pressure is stronger in the right than left arm due to the high velocity jet of blood being directed preferentially into the innominate artery, and there is an easily palpable thrill in the suprasternal notch. In subvalvar stenosis the point of maximal intensity of the systolic murmur will be the third or fourth left intercostal space at the sternal border and differential diagnosis will be from a small ventricular septal defect.

The *chest X-ray* may be normal although post-stenotic dilatation of ascending aorta may be seen. Cardiomegaly will be present only with severe stenosis when prominence of the ascending aorta may be more marked. Calcification of the aortic valve may be seen in older patients but not in children. The *ECG* will be normal when stenosis is mild or moderate. Severe stenosis results in left ventricular hypertrophy as judged from voltage criteria. Eventually T-wave inversion over the left chest or inferior (II, III, aVF) leads will be found. It should be stressed that in contrast to pulmonary stenosis, the *ECG* may be normal when left ventricular outflow tract obstruction is severe. *Echocardiography* may reveal a thickened aortic valve which opens in eccentric fashion, as well as demonstrating left ventricular wall hypertrophy. At *cardiac catheterization* the left ventricle must be entered. Comparison of left ventricular with aortic systolic pressure demonstrates a pressure drop

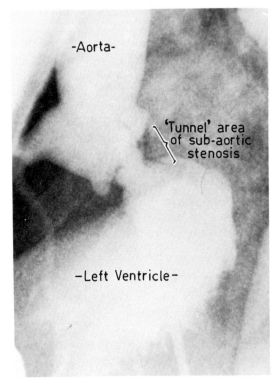

Fig. 34.1 Left ventriculogram in patient with severe aortic stenosis. This patient has sub-valvar and valvar stenosis. The sub-valvar stenosis can be considered an example of tunnel obstruction. (By courtesy of Drs L. M. Bargeron and B. Sota.)

across the aortic valve. A left ventriculogram will demarcate the precise anatomy of the obstruction (Fig. 34.1), and an aortogram should also be performed.

Treatment

Mild stenosis requires no treatment except for antibiotic prophylaxis for dental extractions or planned surgical procedures. Penicillin, or perhaps optimally penicillin and streptomycin, should be administered one hour before the procedure and should be continued for the subsequent three days. If the antibiotic is given earlier, penicillin-resistant organisms will have time to colonize the mouth so that if they were subsequently liberated into the circulation during tooth extraction, penicillin-resistant infective endocarditis could be produced. Aortic valvotomy or some other operation to relieve left ventricular outflow tract obstruction should be performed in all symptomatic patients, those with T-wave changes on *ECG* and in those where the left ventricular systolic pressure is markedly elevated (roughly more than twice aortic). For calcific stenosis, aortic valve replacement will be necessary. Severe aortic stenosis causing heart failure in infants requires emergency valvotomy. Frequently the valve tissue is grossly myxomatous and deformed so that surgery is somewhat unrewarding. The hospital mortality for aortic valvotomy in childhood is 0–5 per cent but in infants ranges from 20–40 per cent.

Subvalvar stenosis can sometimes be relieved directly but tunnel stenosis affords a formidable surgical challenge. Direct relief of obstruction may not be possible so that aortic root replacement with reimplantation of coronary arteries or the insertion of a valved conduit between apex of left ventricle and descending aorta has been advocated.

AORTIC INCOMPETENCE
Trivial aortic incompetence is frequently found with a bicuspid aortic valve. The child will be asymptomatic. On examination abnormal findings will be an ejection click maximal at the apex and a soft early diastolic descrescendo murmur maximal in expiration at the third left intercostal space. Usually, but not invariably, a soft ejection systolic murmur will be heard in the second right intercostal space.

More severe degrees of regurgitation will produce louder murmurs which may merge so as to simulate a continuous murmur maximal in the second or third left intercostal space. The systolic component is due to the increased stroke volume traversing the aortic valve. The patient may have minimal breathlessness on exertion and in addition to the abnormal auscultatory findings will have a prominent apical impulse and bouncing or collapsing pulses. These findings may be present in patients with Marfan's syndrome and dilatation of the aortic root.

The *ECG* shows voltage criteria of left ventricular hypertrophy and the *chest X-ray* some cardiomegaly with dilation of ascending aorta (Fig. 7.4).

In the absence of severe aortic stenosis valve replacement is indicated only when heart failure or severe breathlessness on exertion ensues.

References
Friedman, W. F. and Roberts, W. D. (1966). Vitamin D and the supravalvar aortic

stenosis syndrome. The transplacental effects of vitamin D on the aorta of the rabbit. *Circulation* **34**, 77.

Rowe, R. D. (1972). Stenosis of conducting arteries in infants and children. In *Birth defects*, p. 69. Original Article Series 8 (no. 5).

Seelig, M. S. (1969). Vitamin D and cardiovascular, renal and brain damage in infancy and childhood. *Annals of the New York Academy of Science* **147**, 539.

Shone, J. D., Sellers, R. D., Anderson, R. C., Adams, P., Lillehei, C. W. and Edwards, J. E. (1963). The developmental complex of 'parachute mitral valve', supravalvar ring of left atrium, subaortic stenosis and coarctation of aorta. *American Journal of Cardiology* **11**, 714.

35 Anomalies resulting in a continuous murmur in an acyanotic child

An uncommon but important sign in an asymptomatic or mildly breathless child is the presence of a continuous murmur maximal in the second, third, or fourth intercostal space. The apical impulse and pulse pressure may be normal or increased. That the child does not have cyanotic heart disease is confirmed by arterial blood gas sampling in 100 per cent oxygen. This will exclude pulmonary atresia with ventricular septal defect and systemic-pulmonary collaterals (Chapter 25) and truncal incompetence (Chapter 30) both of which also have a single second sound. The differential diagnosis consists of aortic incompetence (see above), persistent ductus arteriosus (Chapter 32), ventricular septal defect plus aortic incompetence (Chapter 21), aorto-pulmonary window (Chapter 31), ruptured sinus of Valsalva (see below), coronary arteriovenous fistula (see below), aorto-left ventricular tunnel (see below), pulmonary incompetence (absent pulmonary valve syndrome, see below), and peripheral pulmonary stenosis (Chapter 33). Some of these anomalies are rare but will be dealt with briefly for completeness.

Ruptured sinus of Valsalva

Aneurysms of the sinus of Valsalva rupture typically into the right ventricular outflow tract or right atrium. The moment of rupture in older children may be accompanied by severe chest pain although most sinus of Valsalva fistulae are detected because of a basal continuous murmur in an asymptomatic child. Breathlessness occurs if the left-to-right shunt is large. This defect is frequently associated with a ventricular septal defect and/or aortic incompetence. Surgical closure is required especially as the risk of infective endocarditis is high.

Absent pulmonary valve syndrome (congenital pulmonary incompetence)

In this uncommon anomaly the pulmonary valve is represented by ridges of fibromuscular tissue. This may cause pulmonary outflow tract obstruction but pulmonary incompetence dominates and is associated with gross dilatation of the proximal main right and left pulmonary arteries although the distal vessels are normal or small. A subaortic ventricular septal defect is commonly associated. Clinical examination reveals evidence of right ventricular hypertrophy with normal pulses. The second sound is single and a loud to-and-fro murmur which may appear continuous is heard. The *ECG* shows evidence of right ventricular hypertrophy while on *chest X-ray* gross dilatation of the proximal pulmonary vessels is seen. Surgical correction may be complicated by the reduced peripheral pulmonary vascular bed and the mortality at surgery is approximately 30 per cent.

Arteriovenous fistulae

An arteriovenous fistula constitutes an abnormal communication between artery and vein without interposition of a capillary bed. Angiomatous malformations which may be multiple or single form one group and are widespread in patients with multiple hereditary telangiectasia (Osler–Rendu–Weber disease). The commonest example of an abnormal vascular channel is that between a cerebral artery and the great vein of Galen.

Cerebral arteriovenous fistulae (aneurysm of the vein of Galen). This anomaly usually gives rise to neonatal heart failure and signs of pulmonary hypertension and may be associated with coarctation due to abnormal flow distribution in the fetus (see Chapter 4). Bounding carotid pulses will be detected in contrast to poor limb pulses and a cerebral bruit may or may not be heard, although even when present this is not diagnostic. Convulsions may occur. Cardiac catheterization and angiography confirm the diagnosis, high oxygen saturations being found in the superior vena cava with elevated right-sided pressures. Arterial desaturation when present results from right to left shunting across a foramen ovale consequent to increased superior vena caval return. Surgery is usually unsuccessful. In patients surviving the neonatal period hydrocephalus may develop.

Multiple hereditary telangiectasia has a simple dominant mode of transmission affecting males and females equally. Widespread small angiomatous lesions are found in the skin, mucous membranes, liver, kidneys, brain, and sometimes lungs (see below). Haemoptysis, epistaxis, haematuria, rectal, and vaginal bleeding may occur. Either in this condition or as isolated lesions large hepatic haemangiomata can produce high output cardiac failure, with bounding pulses and a hyperdynamic cardiac impulse. Liver function tests may be abnormal. Surgery is largely unsuccessful, the lesions sometimes regress, and both radiotherapy and corticosteroids have been advocated as treatment.

Large arteriovenous fistulae affecting the extremities can produce a swollen hot deformed limb with hypertrophied or deformed bones. High output failure may supervene. The surgical management of these lesions is not considered in this book.

Pulmonary arteriovenous fistulae may be single or multiple and occur between a pulmonary or systemic artery and a pulmonary vein. When there is an abnormal communication between pulmonary artery and vein desaturated blood bypasses the lungs to enter the left side of the heart. Hence there is arterial desaturation and the patient will be cyanosed and clubbed. If there are multiple small pulmonary arteriovenous fistulae no other abnormalities will be found on physical examination. Apart from cardiomegaly the *chest X-ray* will be normal and definitive diagnosis is made by lung biopsy. More commonly there are one or more large angiomatous lesions which can be seen as isolated opacities on the plain *chest X-ray*. On physical examination they may be accompanied by a localized audible bruit. Surgical excision of large lesions should be carried out as haemoptysis, which may be massive, may occur.

Coronary arteriovenous fistulae

This rare anomaly consists of a tortuous dilated vessel arising from a coronary artery and communicating with any of the four cardiac chambers or the pulmonary artery. The fistula usually communicates with the right side of the heart producing a left-to-right shunt. Symptoms depend on the magnitude of the shunt and auscultation reveals a continuous murmur. Surgery is indicated.

Aortic – left ventricular tunnel

Even more uncommon than the preceding anomalies, this endothelialized tunnel has its origin just above a sinus of Valsalva (usually right) and enters the outflow portion of the left ventricle. It simulates signs of aortic incompetence, is diagnosed by an aortogram, and requires surgical closure.

36 Congenital mitral valve anomalies

Prolapsed mitral valve
This clinical syndrome is characterized by posterior protrusion of a mitral valve leaflet during systole. This ballooning of the valve may be due to redundant valve tissue, abnormal chordae tendineae, or papillary muscle dysfunction. Whether a minor degree of prolapse detected by echocardiography or angiocardiography should be considered normal or pathological when the valve is competent is uncertain.

Patients are asymptomatic unless associated arrhythmias produce palpitations. Physical examination reveals a mid-systolic click and late systolic apical murmur although either may be absent. The murmur reflects mitral incompetence and the click accompanies sudden tensing of chordae tendineae or a valve leaflet. In children the *ECG* is usually normal, the T-wave changes in leads II, III, and aVF found in older patients rarely being seen. *Chest X-ray* is unremarkable but the diagnosis can be confirmed on echocardiography (Chapter 9).

Apart from penicillin prophylaxis for dental extractions no treatment is indicated.

Congenital mitral incompetence
When unassociated with myocardial dysfunction or atrioventricular canal defects mitral incompetence is rare, but cleft anterior or posterior mitral valve leaflets have been described as isolated anomalies as has 'an anomalous mitral arcade' as a remediable cause of gross mitral incompetence. When incompetence is severe valve replacement is usually necessary.

Parachute mitral valve
In this anomaly chordae tendineae of both leaflets converge to a single papillary muscle. Congenital mitral stenosis is produced sometimes with mild incompetence. Parachute mitral valve may be associated with a stenosing ring of the left atrium, subaortic stenosis and/or coarctation of the aorta (Shone's syndrome).

Signs of mitral stenosis (Chapter 42) may be produced by parachute valves and by double mitral valve orifices. The various causes of left ventricular inflow obstruction including cor triatriatum can best be differentiated using echocardiography.

References

Daoud, G., Kaplan, S., Perrin, E. V., Dorst, J. G., and Edwards, F. K. (1963). Congenital mitral stenosis. *Circulation* **27**, 185.

Macartney, F. J., Scott, O., Ionescu, M. I., and Deverall, P. B. (1974). Diagnosis and management of parachute mitral valve and supravalvar mitral ring. *British Heart Journal* **36**, 641.

Shone, J. D., Sellers, R. D., Anderson, R. C., Adams, P., Lillehei, C. W., and Edwards, J. E. (1963). The developmental complex of 'parachute mitral valve', supravalvular ring of the left atrium, subaortic stenosis and coarctation of the aorta. *American Journal of Cardiology* **11**, 714.

37 Anomalous origin of coronary arteries from pulmonary trunk

Anomalous origin of the right coronary artery from the pulmonary artery is usually an incidental finding at post-mortem. In contrast, anomalous origin of the left coronary artery from the pulmonary artery usually produces severe symptoms as the artery, although perfused at low pressure, has to supply blood to the left ventricular myocardium. During fetal life the pulmonary artery and aorta are at identical pressures and therefore no haemodynamic disturbance occurs. After birth as the pulmonary vascular resistance, and hence pulmonary artery pressure, falls, the area of myocardium supplied by the left coronary becomes ischaemic (except in a minority of patients who have a well developed collateral circulation supplied by the right coronary artery).

Clinical features
Infants with an anomalous left coronary artery present either with early heart failure or with anginal attacks in which the baby cries, becomes cold and clammy, and looks shocked. If the baby survives these episodes, chronic heart failure with a dilated left ventricle and functional mitral incompetence may ensue. The ECG may show evidence of myocardial infarction with deep Q-waves and inverted T-waves in leads I, AVL and the left chest leads, possibly with ST segment elevation. In other patients left sided T-wave inversion is the sole abnormality. Cardiac catheterization and angiography confirm the diagnosis. A small left-to-right shunt may be detected at pulmonary arterial level, flow occurring through the right coronary artery via collaterals to the anomalous left coronary artery. Root aortograms fail to identify a left coronary artery while selective right coronary arteriography will show retrograde filling of the left coronary.

Treatment
In the past, ligation of the left coronary artery at its origin from the pulmonary trunk has been performed but this may lead to myocardial infarction. Recently good results have been achieved by direct anas-

tomosis of the anomalous coronary artery plus a sleeve of pulmonary artery to the aorta or by creation of an aorto-pulmonary window through which the left coronary is patched into the aorta.

References

Bland, E. F., White, P. D., and Garland, J. (1933). Congenital anomalies of the coronary arteries. *American Heart Journal* **8**, 787.

Lurie, P. R. (1978). Abnormalities and diseases of the Coronary Vessels. In *Heart disease in infants, children and adolescents* (ed. A. J. Moss, F. H. Adams, and G. C. Emmanouiltides), 2nd edn. Williams and Wilkins, Baltimore.

38 Coarctation of the aorta

Anatomy and embryology
Coarctation can be considered in two main forms which may co-exist, namely juxtaductal coarctation or tubular hypoplasia (Fig. 38.1). In older children isolated juxtaductal coarctation is frequently caused by an indentation of the posterior aortic wall opposite the ductus

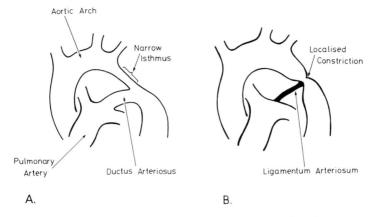

Fig. 38.1 The difference between tubular hypoplasia (A) and juxtaductal coarctation (B) of the aortic arch.

arteriosus. In some infants the aortic isthmus has been shown to insert not into the descending aorta but into the distal part of the ductus so that subsequent ductal constriction produces obstruction. Tubular narrowing of the aortic isthmus is the consequence of reduced aortic flow in the fetus and is frequently associated with intracardiac anomalies resulting in left-sided obstruction or preferential main pulmonary artery flow (see Chapter 4a).

Incidence
Coarctation is the commonest primary cardiovascular cause of heart failure in an acyanotic neonate in the first week of life. It is frequently associated with both acyanotic and cyanotic heart disease in this age group. In older children it is a relatively common type of acyanotic congenital cardiovascular anomaly.

Clinical findings

Presentation
Older children or adults are usually asymptomatic, being diagnosed as a result of evaluation of a heart murmur heard at incidental examination, because of absent or reduced femoral pulses, or because of the finding of upper limb hypertension during routine or insurance examination. Hypertensive encephalopathy is rarely the presenting feature.

Physical examination
Infants, as indicated, may present with early heart failure, but many are diagnosed because of absent or grossly reduced femoral pulses. This latter feature is the cardinal sign of coarctation and the disparity between upper and lower limb pressures should be confirmed by measurement of the blood pressure in both right and left arms, as well as in the legs. This is best achieved, at least in infants, using the Doppler technique. It must be remembered that up to 20 mmHg systolic pressure difference between upper and lower limbs is a normal finding in the neonate (because of isthmal narrowing). Other features sometimes found on examination are left ventricular hypertrophy, continuous murmurs maximal over the scapulae resulting from flow through collateral vessels, basal ejection systolic murmurs, and an ejection click. It should be stressed that coarctation, especially in infancy, frequently accompanies other cardiac anomalies, but never those where blood is shunted away from the main pulmonary artery into the aorta. Such a flow distribution in the fetus is incompatible with aortic narrowing. Furthermore, coarctation will not be manifest at birth as the ductus arteriosus offers a conduit bypassing the site of potential obstruction. It is only with ductal closure that a pressure difference develops between upper and lower limbs.

The *chest X-ray* shows cardiomegaly in the presence of heart failure when coarctation is severe. The rounded convexity of the aortic knuckle may be indented at the site of coarctation. Rib notching will be observed when a collateral circulation has been established for some time. The *ECG* shows left ventricular hypertrophy or is normal. In infants right ventricular hypertrophy may dominate, although this latter finding is perhaps more typical of an interrupted aortic arch, the other anomaly which is associated with reduced femoral pulses. Right ventricular hypertrophy is also found when there are additional anomalies such as a VSD with pulmonary hypertension. *Cardiac*

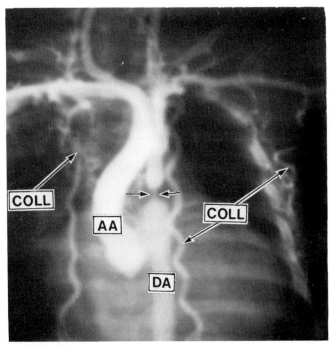

Fig. 38.2 Frontal projection of an aortogram performed in a patient with severe isolated juxtaductal coarctation. Prominent internal mammary vessels are seen, which act as collaterals.

catheterization should be performed to demarcate the anatomy (Fig. 38.2) and ascertain the presence of any associated intracardiac anomalies. In older children when right and left arm pressures are equal and raised, catheterization is sometimes deemed unnecessary as obstruction must be distal to the left subclavian artery.

Treatment
Coarctation causing heart failure or symptoms in infancy must be relieved surgically as a matter of urgency. Asymptomatic coarctation with any significant hypertension should also be resected at any time after six months of age, and this should carry a negligible mortality. If significant coarctation is not treated early, hypertension in upper and lower limbs may persist, despite adequate relief of obstruction.

When coarctation is the isthmal narrowing (preductal) variety, apart from mortality due to associated intracardiac anomalies, it may be technically difficult to remove or bypass all obstruction to aortic flow.

Especially if there is in addition a hypoplastic aortic arch, surgical mortality is high.

Classical resection of the coarcted area and end-to-end anastomosis has been superseded in infancy by a technique which allows angioplastic repair of the narrowed area, using the patient's subclavian artery. This vessel is divided and turned down to form a side-to-side onlay graft. The principal complication of resection of coarctation in infancy has in the past been that of re-coarctation (10 per cent). Angioplastic repair is a definite advance in the treatment of coarctation in these young patients.

Treatment of coarctation of the aorta in older children can be effectively carried out by resection and end-to-end anastomosis. Occasionally a long hypoplastic segment is present, which precludes end-to-end anastomosis, and in this case interposition of a Dacron tube prosthesis can be carried out. The hospital mortality for this condition is 0–5 per cent.

References

Ho, S. Y. and Anderson, R. H. (1979). Coarctation, tubular hypoplasia and the ductus arteriosus: a histological study of 35 specimens. *British Heart Journal* **41**, 268.

Rudolph, A. M., Heymann, M. A., and Spitznas, U. (1972). Hemodynamic considerations in the development of narrowing of the aorta. *American Journal of Cardiology* **30**, 514.

Shinebourne, E. A., Tam, A. S. Y., Elseed, A. M., Parneth, M., Lennox, S. C., Cleland, W. P., Lincoln, C., Joseph, M. C., and Anderson, R. H. (1976). Coarctation of the aorta in infancy and childhood. *British Heart Journal* **38**, 375.

Sinha, S. N., Kardatzke, M. L. Cole, R. B., Muster, A. J., Wessel, H. U., and Paul, M. H. (1969). Coarctation of the aorta in infancy. *Circulation* **40**, 385.

Waldhausen, J. A. and Nahrwold, D. L. (1966). Repair of coarctation of the aorta with a subclavian flap. *Journal of Thoracic and Cardiovascular Surgery* **51**, 532.

39 Interrupted aortic arch

Anatomy

The anomaly is classified on the precise site of interruption of the arch. Most commonly the interruption is immediately distal to the left sub-clavian artery, but it can be distal to the left common carotid or to the innominate (brachiocephalic) artery. Lower limb blood supply is maintained via the ductus arteriosus. Interruption of the aortic arch is unusual as an isolated entity. Frequently co-existent subaortic stenosis associated with a malalignment ventricular septal defect has caused reduced antegrade aortic flow during fetal development. Interrupted aortic arch can also accompany truncus arteriosus (see Chapter 30) or aortopulmonary window.

Clinical findings

Patients present usually as young neonates with signs identical to that of severe coarctation. As the ductus closes, severe metabolic acidosis develops due to hypoperfusion of the lower body, and the patients become extremely ill. Apart from reduced or absent femoral pulses, there will be signs of pulmonary hypertension. Marked right ventricular hypertrophy on ECG in a patient with signs of coarctation alerts one to the possibility of arch interruption. The diagnosis is made by angiography.

Treatment

As an emergency procedure, infusion of prostaglandin E_1 or E_2 to dilate the ductus arteriosus can allow correction of profound metabolic acidosis, which may otherwise be impossible. Symptomatic improvement should be followed by urgent surgical intervention, probably best carried out using profound hypothermia and circulatory arrest. This has resulted in survival of a number of these patients. Successful treatment depends upon reconstruction of the arch of the aorta. This can be performed by means of an interposition graft or by using the ductus arteriosus as an autologous tube graft. The condition still remains one of the most challenging encountered in all surgery of congenital heart disease, and the mortality is high.

References

Celoria, G. C. and Patten, R. B. (1959). Congenital absence of the aortic arch. *American Heart Journal* **58**, 407.

Van Praagh, R. Bernhard, W. P., Rosenthal, A., Parisi, L. F., and Fyler, D. C. (1971). Interrupted aortic arch: surgical treatment. *American Journal of Cardiology* **27**, 200.

40 Vascular rings and aortic arch anomalies

Anatomy and embryology

Vascular rings constitute anomalies of the aortic arches and their derivatives which result in compression of the trachea and/or oesophagus. The precise embryology and anatomy of these anomalies has been excellently summarized by Stewart, Kincaid, and Edwards (1964), and will not be considered here. Anomalies of clinical importance are a right aortic arch with left ligamentum arteriosum or persistent ductus arteriosus, a double aortic arch, abnormal position of the innominate artery, aberrant right subclavian artery, and anomalous left pulmonary artery arising from the right side of the main pulmonary artery.

Clinical findings

An aberrant right subclavian artery as an isolated anomaly rarely causes symptoms, but may cause difficulty in swallowing (dysphagia lusoria). The other vascular rings in addition cause stridor, which may be severe, wheezing, and recurrent chest infections. Lobar emphysema may complicate partial bronchial obstruction.

In order to minimize tracheal compression, the child may exhibit marked hyperextension of the neck. The heart will be normal to examination as will be the ECG. Plain *chest X-ray* will demonstrate a right aortic arch when present, and may show a mediastinal mass resulting from an aberrant left pulmonary artery.

Diagnosis can be made by barium swallow. With a double aortic arch bilateral concave indentations are seen in the frontal projection at the levels of the arches, similar findings being present with a right arch and left ductus arteriosus. In both these cases, lateral views show the oesophagus to be compressed from behind, whereas an anomalous left pulmonary artery compresses the front of the oesophagus as it passes from right to left between it and the trachea. *Angiography* will be necessary to identify other anomalies, and provides optimal confirmation of the anatomy.

Treatment

In all these anomalies the object of treatment is to relieve the constricting ring compressing the trachea and oesophagus. All anomalies can be treated through a left thoracotomy. When there is a right arch with a left ductus or ligament it is only necessary to divide the persistent ductus or ligamentum, thus breaking the constricting ring. In double aortic arch, there is a minor and a major arch; the major arch usually gives rise to the head vessels. Division of the minor arch can be safely performed.

When the innominate artery is abnormally displaced to the left of the trachea it may compress it anteriorly. Treatment consists of suspending the innominate artery from the back of the sternum, thereby lifting it off the trachea. An anomalous right subclavian artery is rarely symptomatic, although it can cause symptoms in later life. Division of the subclavian artery as it arises from the first part of the descending thoracic aorta relieves any oesophageal constriction.

References

Lincoln, J. C. R., Deverall, P. B., Stark, J., Aberdeen, E., and Waterston, D. J. (1969). Vascular anomalies compressing the oesophagus and trachea. *Thorax* **24**, 295.

Stewart, J. R., Kincaid, O. W., and Edwards, J. E. (1964). *An atlas of vascular rings and related malformations of the aortic arch system.* Charles C. Thomas, Springfield, Ill.

41 Hypertrophic cardiomyopathy and fibroelastosis

HYPERTROPHIC OBSTRUCTIVE CARDIOMYOPATHY
(Idiopathic hypertrophic subaortic stenosis)

Anatomy and pathology
The heart shows asymmetrical hypertrophy of the left ventricle and less commonly of the right ventricle. The interventricular septum is particularly involved and may bulge into the cavities of both left and right ventricles. The cavity of the left ventricle may be grossly reduced in size. Variable obstruction to left ventricular emptying is produced during systole by apposition of the anterior leaflet of the mitral valve to the hypertrophied septum. On histology, areas of myocardium are found where the muscle cell bundles are disorganized with abnormal orientation of myofibril and myofilaments. Such areas can also be found in hearts exhibiting secondary hypertrophy due to, for example, aortic stenosis, and the full significance of the histological changes remains to be established.

Incidence
A strong familial incidence has been reported but the majority of cases occur sporadically. The condition may present in infancy but more commonly symptoms first occur in the third or fourth decade. An association with Pompe's disease and Friedrich's ataxia has been noted and a syndrome of multiple lentigenoses, hypertrophic obstructive cardiomyopathy, and intellectual impairment is described.

Clinical features
Many patients are asymptomatic, although infants may present with heart failure and older patients with fatiguability, syncope, breathlessness, or angina. In the older group symptoms are no more marked in those with demonstrable obstruction to left ventricular emptying than in those without and symptoms appear to depend on impaired left ventricular filling.

Physical examination shows a rapid upstroke but normal or low volume pulse. The apical impulse as well as the pulse may be double and on auscultation a systolic murmur can be heard at the lower left sternal border.

ECG shows voltage criteria of left ventricular hypertrophy, deep left-sided Q-waves are found and later T-waves become inverted. Features simulating the Wolff–Parkinson–White are common with a short P–R interval and delta wave. Cardiomegaly may be seen on *chest X-ray*.

Definitive diagnosis can be made using *echocardiography* (see Chapter 9), which demonstrates a thickened interventricular septum, small left ventricular cavity, and abnormal systolic anterior movement of the anterior cusp of the mitral valve.

At *cardiac catheterization* systolic gradients may be found between left ventricle and aorta and between right ventricle and pulmonary artery. The gradient is increased by isoprenaline. Angiography confirms the anatomical and echocardiographic features.

Treatment
Propranolol or other beta adrenergic blocking agents are used as first-line therapy in symptomatic patients. Myotomy with myomec-tomy also has an important part to play in relieving symptoms although whether this increases longevity is uncertain.

ENDOCARDIAL FIBROELASTOSIS
Pathology
Endocardial fibroelastosis may be isolated or accompany congenital anomalies such as the hypoplastic left heart syndrome, aortic stenosis, or coarctation. Although usually sporadic, it may be familial. It consists of gross thickening of endocardial and sub-endocardial regions of the left ventricle, and sometimes left atrium. Excess elastin and collagen is deposited and the endocardial surface appears pale and opaque. It is probable that endocardial fibroelastosis represents the pathological response to a variety of abnormal stimuli, but the precise aetiology is unknown.

Clinical findings
Heart failure in an acyanotic infant is how most cases present. Differential diagnosis is principally from myocarditis, congenital mitral incompetence, paroxysmal supraventricular tachycardia, or from the other left-sided anomalies with which it may, in any case, be

associated. Auscultation reveals a third heart sound and possibly the murmur of functional mitral incompetence. The *chest X-ray* shows cardiomegaly with pulmonary venous congestion. The *ECG* shows characteristic T-wave inversion over the left chest leads, usually with abnormally large left ventricular voltages (Fig. 8.3).

The diagnosis of primary left ventricular dysfunction can be easily confirmed echocardiographically, although endocardial fibroelastosis cannot be distinguished in this way from neonatal myocarditis or certain other non-hypertrophic cardiomyopathies.

Treatment

There is no specific treatment but digoxin and diuretics should be given to treat heart failure. Many patients, especially those with a positive family history, die in infancy. Other children show decreasing heart size over several years and appear to be recovering, although without cardiac biopsy the diagnosis in these children is circumstantial. When endocardial fibroelastosis appears to accompany symptomatic coarctation, it is always worthwhile resecting the coarctation, as striking improvement may follow. In such cases left ventricular dysfunction is in part due to subendocardial ischaemia, the high end-diastolic pressure in the ventricle, and shortening of diastole due to tachycardia, resulting in decreased myocardial perfusion.

References

Buckley, B. H. (1977). Idiopathic hypertrophic subaortic stenosis afflicted: Idols of the cave and the marketplace. *American Journal of Cardiology* **40**, 476.

Keith, J. D., Rose, V., and Manning, J. A. (1978). Endocardial fibroelastosis. In *Heart disease in infancy and childhood* (ed. J. D. Keith, R. D. Rowe, and P. Vlad), 3rd edn. Macmillan, London.

Maron, B. J., Henry, W. L., Clark, C. E., Redwood, D. R., Roberts, W. C., and Epstein, S. E. (1976). Asymetric septal hypertrophy in childhood. *Circulation* **53**, 9.

Teare, D. (1958). Asymmetrical hypertrophy of the heart in young adults. *British Heart Journal* **20**, 1.

42 Rheumatic fever and rheumatic heart disease

Incidence and aetiology
While rheumatic fever has become extremely uncommon in many developed countries, in those that are underdeveloped it remains the major cause of cardiac disability in older children and young adults. Thus, children with acute or chronic rheumatic heart disease will always be found in the University Hospital, Khartoum while at Brompton Hospital no British child with this condition has been seen during the last six years.

Socioeconomic factors play a major part in these differences. Poverty, large families with overcrowding, and poor housing predispose to recurrent cross infection. In particular, repeated infections with beta haemolytic streptococci are facilitated. There is no evidence to indicate that the virulence of the causative organism, Lancefield Group A beta haemolytic streptococcus, varies in different parts of the world. Similarly no differences in host susceptibility have as yet been firmly demonstrated between different ethnic groups. It is of note that in those countries where the incidence of rheumatic fever is now very low the decline in incidence had started before the introduction of penicillin and other antimicrobial agents. This again lays emphasis on the importance of socioeconomic factors in aetiology of the disease and this must be taken into account if the incidence of rheumatic fever is to be reduced in developing countries. Rheumatic fever affects mostly older children, being uncommon in children under five and rare in those under two years of age.

Pathogenesis
The Lancefield Group A haemolytic streptococcus is the causative organism of rheumatic fever but the specific mechanisms producing the pathological lesions are not known. Autoimmune mechanisms have been invoked but not proven. There is no definite evidence that viruses play a role in the disease. While streptococcal infections are common only a small proportion of infected individuals develop rheumatic fever. Infections of tonsils or pharynx precede acute rheumatic fever in a high proportion of cases but streptococcal skin infections are not followed by rheumatic fever although frequently preceding acute glomerulonephritis.

Microbiology of Lancefield group A beta haemolytic streptococcus
This single-celled organism has a capsule of hyaluronate which
encloses a three-layered cell wall consisting, from without, of a protein
layer, a carbohydrate layer, and an inner layer; the cell wall in turn
surrounds a central core of cytoplasm. The most important wall protein
is that termed M protein to which antiphagocytic activity is related, as
is the virulence of the organism. Differences in the carbohydrate layer
determine the serological varieties of the organism. Group A strains
produce most infection in man. Group A streptococci secrete many
substances into the surrounding tissues. Among the most important
are streptolysin O, streptokinase, hyaluronidase, and erythrogenic
toxin, which causes the rash of scarlet fever. Antibodies against streptolysin O can be easily quantitated and are most commonly measured
(antistreptolysin O titre, ASO titre) as evidence of previous streptococcal infection. These antibodies can usually be detected a week
after an untreated infection and reach a maximum in three to five
weeks. Higher ASO titres are usually but not always found in subjects
who develop rheumatic fever. Of note is the observation that the ASO
titres rise more after streptococcal throat infections than after streptococcal skin infections.

Clinical features of acute rheumatic fever usually occur two to three
weeks after streptococcal throat infection but latent periods of as little
as five days or as long as six weeks occur. Some patients have no
previous history of streptococcal infection while others are asymptomatic carriers.

Pathology
The acute rheumatic process involves the myocardium, endocardium,
and pericardium. The Aschoff-body is pathognomonic of rheumatic
fever, usually but not always indicating acute rheumatic activity. It
consists of a central perivascular necrotic core surrounded by a rosette
of large cells with basophilic cytoplasm and polymorphous nuclei.
Later the Aschoff-bodies become converted to healed scars and they
may result in extensive myocardial fibrosis, cardiac dilatation, and
secondary hypertrophy. Rheumatic endocarditis results in oedema and
an inflammatory reaction in the leaflets and chordae tendineae. Warty
vegetations are found where the leaflets are apposed. Subsequent
thickening, deformation, and shortening of the chordae and retraction
and fusion of the valve leaflets leads to grossly deformed valves.
Left-sided valves are affected far more commonly than those on the
right side, mitral valve disease being the commonest. Rheumatic

pericarditis is common but haemodynamically important pericardial effusions are uncommon.

ACUTE RHEUMATIC FEVER

Clinical findings

Presentation
Clinical presentation is variable but children usually present with manifestations of rheumatic arthritis, carditis, or chorea. In under-developed countries children nearly always present late in the course of their illness and rarely present with minor symptoms such as arthralgia or skin rashes. The five to fifteen-year-old age group is most commonly affected with an equal sex incidence. A preceding history of sore throat may be elicited in approximately half the children.

Flitting severe arthritis affecting large joints such as knees, ankles, or elbows is a common mode of presentation especially in older children. The joint is swollen, painful, hot and tender for three to ten days before it gradually subsides and typically another joint becomes involved. During this time the child is febrile, ill, and complains of generalized aches and pains. Small joints, spine, hips, and shoulders are rarely affected while those joints that are involved recover completely.

Severe carditis presents as heart failure with breathlessness and possibly palpitations as prominent symptoms. Chest pain more marked on inspiration may accompany pericarditis. Examination reveals an ill child with fever, pallor, marked tachycardia, and elevated jugular venous pressure. The pulse may be collapsing because of fever, anaemia or aortic incompetence, singly or in combination. As many of the children in underdeveloped countries will be thin, marked precordial pulsations are seen. Auscultation reveals soft heart sounds, a gallop rhythm (third heart sound), and typically a soft apical pansystolic murmur due to mitral incompetence. There may be a pericardial friction rub. An apical mid-diastolic murmur (Carey Coombs) due to increased flow across the mitral valve is less common. The soft early diastolic murmur of aortic incompetence may also be heard maximally at the third left intercostal space.

Rheumatic (Sydenham's) chorea is commoner in girls and is usually an isolated manifestation of rheumatic activity. It consists of involuntary, non-repetitive movements of the face, tongue, and limbs. The attacks may last up to six months during which the child has difficulty holding things, writing, and walking. There is emotional lability and hypotonia that may be so severe that the child is bedridden. Dysarthria can be found with involuntary movements of the tongue as a prominent feature. Sometimes only one side of the body is involved (hemichorea).

During episodes of chorea there is conspicuous absence of other manifestations of acute rheumatic fever. In particular, arthritis, carditis, fever, and a high ESR are absent. On a subsequent occasion, however, the child may present with acute rheumatic carditis or arthritis. Fever, which accompanies carditis and arthritis but rarely chorea, is not seen as the sole presenting feature, and subsides when other manifestations of rheumatic fever disappear. Arthralgia in the absence of arthritis is common, as is abdominal pain. Erythema marginatum (a transient, raised, non-pruritic, clearly demarcated red macular rash with normal skin colour in its centre usually involving the lower limbs and trunk) is uncommon and can be found in other diseases. It is more easily seen in fair- than dark-skinned children. Rheumatic nodules (painless, sub-cutaneous lesions typically seen on extensor joint surfaces such as elbows and knees) are also uncommon. In contrast, epistaxis is common in rheumatic fever but has many other causes. The American Heart Association has issued guidelines for the diagnosis of rheumatic fever on the basis of major and minor manifestations. These do not seem to be quite as useful in underdeveloped countries where rheumatic fever is most common.

Physical examination

The *chest X-ray* may show varying signs of cardiomegaly depending on the severity of myocarditis. Upper lobe blood diversion or frank pulmonary oedema will accompany congestive heart failure especially with mitral incompetence. Transient cotton wool shadowing in the lungs is rare but may reflect rheumatic pneumonitis.

The *ECG* most commonly shows sinus tachycardia with or without a prolonged P–R interval (first degree block). Atrial fibrillation usually reflects chronic rheumatic heart disease. Large left-sided voltages are sometimes seen but T-waves usually remain upright in V_6, V_7 unless there is overt pericarditis.

The *erythrocyte sedimentation rate* (ESR) is raised in acute rheumatic fever even when the child is in heart failure (which tends to lower the ESR). In the absence of a raised ESR the diagnosis of an active rheumatic process is highly unlikely (except with chorea). The ASO titre, as mentioned previously, is usually elevated during an attack of acute rheumatic fever and tends to remain elevated for some time.

In a patient with signs of mitral or aortic valve disease and fever, bacterial endocarditis must be excluded. The child with a big heart and signs of mitral incompetence may have left ventricular muscle disease (congestive cardiomyopathy), endocardial fibroelastosis (usually affecting a younger age group), or viral myocarditis. T-wave inversion in the electrocardiogram over the left chest leads would suggest a primary myocardial disease. Severe anaemia is a common cause of heart failure in underdeveloped countries and must be excluded.

Treatment
Bed rest is traditionally prescribed for acute rheumatic carditis although its efficacy remains unproven. The pain of acute rheumatic arthritis usually causes the child himself to take to his bed. A ten-day course of penicillin should be routinely given to eradicate residual streptococci. In an ill child this should be administered by intramuscular injection in a dose of 0.5–1 megaunit procaine penicillin daily. Oral administration may be used after a few days in compliant children when adequate supervision is available, although in those countries where rheumatic fever is common this is often not the case. It is also of note that parenteral penicillin is cheaper than oral penicillin.

Heart failure is treated with rest, digoxin, diuretics, and judicious correction of severe anaemia with packed cells. In the majority of children these measures alone will prove effective. Rheumatic arthritis if present is treated with salicylates 100 mg/kg/day in divided doses reducing to 50 or 75 mg/kg/day for three to four weeks. This anti-inflammatory regime provides symptomatic relief of arthritis and fever. Salicylates are also usually given for acute carditis without cardiomegaly but essentially this is to treat the accompanying fever.

If an ill child with acute rheumatic carditis and significant cardiomegaly fails to respond to the measures already outlined the question of steroids must be considered. There is some but by no means conclusive evidence that administration of a short course (two weeks) of prednisone in a dose of 2–3 mg/kg in divided doses over 24 hours may accelerate recovery when the heart is enlarged. In severely ill children steroids may be life saving. Against this, especially in the poorer countries, the risk of activating tuberculosis is high.

Prophylaxis
As the beta haemolytic streptococcus has remained faithfully sensitive to penicillin, long term penicillin prophylaxis at least to the age of 20 years but probably for life is indicated. Either monthly injections of 0.6–1.2 megaunits benzathine penicillin or 125 mg twice daily oral penicillin are effective. Where compliance cannot be certain and cost

of drugs relative to income is high long-acting intramuscular penicillin is preferable. Erythromycin is probably the best alternative for penicillin-sensitive patients but sulphonamides are cheaper, if far less effective.

Prognosis

Especially in poorer countries there is still a significant mortality from acute rheumatic fever, probably compounded by the presence of additional infections, malnutrition, and anaemia. Recurrent attacks are greatly reduced if not abolished by penicillin prophylaxis but socioeconomic factors still dominate the outlook for a child who has had an episode of rheumatic fever.

CHRONIC RHEUMATIC HEART DISEASE

Although many patients will give a history of arthritis, carditis, or chorea, absence of a history of acute rheumatic fever in no way precludes the diagnosis of chronic rheumatic heart disease. Conversely, valvar lesions may be expected in children with a history of recurrent attacks of rheumatic fever.

The mitral valve is affected three times as commonly as the aortic valve. Both valves may be affected and rarely isolated rheumatic aortic incompetence is found in children. Aortic stenosis in childhood is almost always congenital. The tricuspid and pulmonary valves are rarely if ever directly damaged by the rheumatic process although functional tricuspid or even pulmonary incompetence may accompany heart failure due to left-sided lesions.

Mitral stenosis

Although severe rheumatic mitral stenosis will not be found in children from the developed world, severe stenosis is not uncommon in underdeveloped countries and may be seen in children as young as five or six years of age. Girls are affected more commonly than boys. Isolated mitral stenosis is less common than combined mitral stenosis and incompetence.

A history of easy fatiguability, palpitations, and breathlessness on exertion are usually the presenting features although the disease process has progressed so far in some children that they present with orthopnoea and pulmonary oedema.

On examination the child may be small for age. Pulses are normal or of reduced volume and there is no cyanosis. The jugular venous pressure may be elevated, and if there is secondary tricuspid incompetence a prominent V-wave will be seen. The first sound may be palpable as may the pulmonary component of the second sound. A left parasternal heave with or without a localized apical diastolic thrill can be felt. The first sound is loud due to the mitral valve closing from a fully opened position secondary to the high left atrial pressure. The pulmonary component of the second sound is loud. There may be an opening snap after the second sound if the mitral valve leaflets remain mobile. A low pitched rumbling mid-diastolic murmur localized to the apex indicates turbulent flow through the narrowed mitral valve orifice. Presystolic accentuation may be heard in patients who are in sinus rhythm (accompanying atrial systole, 'A'-wave) but is lost in atrial fibrillation. When mitral stenosis becomes very severe the murmur disappears and the children present with signs of pulmonary hypertension plus a loud first heart sound. Under such circumstances the early diastolic murmur of pulmonary incompetence (Graham–Steel) may be heard.

Diagnosis is made by the use of echocardiography (see Chapter 9) and in isolated mitral stenosis cardiac catheterization should not be necessary.

Complications
Severe mitral stenosis should always be considered in the differential diagnosis of pulmonary hypertension. Atrial fibrillation occurs but is uncommon in children. Embolic phenomena, usually neurological, may then appear.

Treatment
Acute or chronic heart failure must first be treated with digoxin, diuretics, oxygen, and if necessary morphine. Associated anaemia should be corrected.

The indications for surgery are heart failure, orthopnoea, severe breathlessness on exertion, or other significant symptoms. Elective closed mitral valvotomy should be carried out in children with severe isolated mitral stenosis. Unfortunately, in those parts of the world where this operation is most needed, surgical, nursing, and other facilities are often not locally available.

Mitral incompetence
Despite the relatively early occurrence of mitral stenosis, in many underdeveloped countries mitral incompetence remains the most common cardiac lesion in children with rheumatic heart disease.

Clinical findings

In many patients an apical pansystolic murmur with selective radiation towards the axilla may be heard during presentation with acute rheumatic fever. Most commonly, however, children present with breathlessness of varying severity.

On physical examination the peripheral pulses are normal and precordial bulging may be present in children with severe and longstanding disease. The apex, heaving in nature, is displaced downwards and outwards. The pulmonary component of the second heart sound may be normal or loud in intensity, and an apical third heart sound may be heard. A harsh apical pansystolic murmur of varying intensity is heard at the axilla and below the left scapula.

The *ECG* may be normal or it may reveal the presence of broad and bifid P-waves indicating left atrial hypertrophy. Left ventricular hypertrophy leads to tall R-waves in leads V_5 and V_6 and/or to a deep S-wave in lead V_1. T-wave changes are much less commonly seen, and when present in children with mitral incompetence, the aetiology is more likely to be primary myocardial disease (e.g. congestive cardiomyopathy) than rheumatic. The presence of pulmonary hypertension in children with mitral incompetence does not usually lead to ECG evidence of right ventricular hypertrophy.

On *chest X-ray* the heart size and pulmonary vascular markings may be normal, but with increasing severity of regurgitation, enlargement of the left atrium and an increase in the transverse diameter of the heart may be seen. The left main bronchus is then displaced upwards, the left atrial appendage is more prominent and a double shadow to the right heart border reflects left atrial enlargement occurring posteriorly and to the right. Upper lobe blood diversion may then also be seen.

Mitral incompetence due to causes other than rheumatic fever is frequent in underdeveloped countries. Heart muscle disease, in particular congestive cardiomyopathy, can cause mitral incompetence. Children with the congestive type of cardiomyopathy and mitral incompetence are more ill than children with rheumatic mitral incompetence. They present with severe congestive heart failure and their course is more acutely downhill. The *ECG* tends to show T-wave changes right from the first presentation, which is unusual in patients with rheumatic mitral incompetence. Similarly, the *chest X-ray* reveals gross cardiac enlargement with marked dilatation of the left atrium.

Mitral incompetence may also be seen as an isolated congenital anomaly or as part of an atrioventricular canal defect.

The prolapsed mitral valve syndrome is another cause of mitral incompetence. The murmur in patients with this condition tends to be mid-or late systolic with a mid-systolic click and echocardiography is of great help in distinguishing this entity from rheumatic mitral incompetence.

In any child with mitral incompetence it is important to determine the aetiology since long term prophylaxis with penicillin is indicated only in patients with rheumatic mitral incompetence. Frequently prophylaxis is withheld from such patients because they are thought to have congenital mitral incompetence and this is especially so when patients develop rheumatic fever in early childhood. Conversely, it is not uncommon to find patients with non-rheumatic mitral incompetence unnecessarily maintained on long term prophylaxis. The situation with short term prophylaxis also needs to be clarified since it is frequently not realized that patients with rheumatic mitral incompetence need to receive, in addition to the long term prophylaxis, antibiotic cover shortly before and for some time after minor surgical procedures such as circumcision and tooth extraction.

Apart from management of congestive heart failure, mitral valve replacement or open repair on full cardiopulmonary bypass is the only procedure that can be advised in children with severe mitral incompetence and poor response to medical treatment. The relatively high cost and technical expertise needed to perform this operation as well as the difficulty of adequate post-operative follow-up must be taken into consideration before patients in underdeveloped countries are advised regarding this operation. Furthermore, the risk of recurrence of acute rheumatic carditis is always significant and we have seen patients who, following mitral commissurotomy for rheumatic mitral stenosis, developed acute rheumatic fever with carditis.

Aortic incompetence
Isolated aortic incompetence of rheumatic origin is uncommon. More commonly the findings of aortic incompetence are detected while examining patients presenting with the features of mitral valve disease as described earlier, or during presentation with acute rheumatic fever. When mild, isolated aortic incompetence causes no symptoms. As the condition becomes more severe, breathlessness and palpitations develop, and in patients with mitral valve disease development of aortic incompetence greatly increases the severity of breathlessness and other manifestations of heart failure.

Physical examination usually reveals the presence of collapsing peripheral pulses and prominent arterial pulsations in the neck (Corrigan's sign). The apex is heaving and displaced outwards and downwards. In isolated aortic incompetence the heart sounds are normal in intensity. An early soft diastolic murmur is usually best heard in the third left intercostal space and may also be audible at the apex and second right intercostal space. Using the diaphragm of the stethoscope and listening while the patient is sitting up, and leaning forward, in held expiration makes it less difficult to hear this murmur which is easily missed because of its soft nature. A mid-systolic murmur, usually short and localized to the base of the heart, is frequently heard. In most patients this murmur is due to increased flow of blood through the aortic valve rather than to aortic stenosis.

The ECG may be normal although voltage criteria of left ventricular hypertrophy may be present, especially in children with both aortic and mitral incompetence. Left-sided T-wave changes are uncommon.

In patients with mild aortic incompetence the chest X-ray is normal although a prominent ascending aorta is present with haemodynamically significant incompetence. Increased cardiothoracic diameter due to left ventricular dilatation is seen in patients with severe aortic incompetence. Such patients usually have severe rheumatic mitral valve disease, and the X-ray changes already described for this condition would then be present in addition.

Children who come to hospital in heart failure usually respond to medical treatment with digoxin and diuretics, although in underdeveloped countries their symptoms tend to recur shortly after discharge from hospital. Children with severe aortic incompetence usually have mitral valve disease as well and their symptoms respond poorly to medical treatment. In such patients surgery would mean replacement of both mitral and aortic valves and the same considerations which have been mentioned regarding mitral valve replacement would then hold. The prognosis of mild aortic incompetence is good providing there are no further attacks of acute rheumatic carditis or infective endocarditis.

Aortic stenosis
In children aortic stenosis is rarely caused by rheumatic fever and more commonly is congenital in origin. When present in patients with rheumatic fever, it always accompanies one or more valvar lesions already described. The presence of small peripheral pulses and evidence of left ventricular hypertrophy without dilatation should draw attention to this lesion.

Tricuspid and pulmonary valve involvement

These valves are rarely directly affected by rheumatic fever. Tricuspid incompetence is usually functional in origin and accompanies cardiac dilatation. Its clinical manifestations are a prominent V-wave in the jugular venous pulse, a pansystolic murmur louder on inspiration maximal at the fourth right intercostal space, and a pulsatile enlarged liver.

Tricuspid stenosis can be caused by rheumatic fever but this is rare. Functional pulmonary incompetence is sometimes present in patients with pulmonary hypertension, manifest as an early diastolic murmur maximal at the second left intercostal space.

Reference

Markowitz, N. and Gordis, L. (1972). *Rheumatic Fever*, 2nd edition. W. B. Saunders, Philadelphia.

43 Infective endocarditis

Incidence and aetiology
Bacterial endocarditis is uncommon in infants or young children with congenital heart disease, being more frequently found in older children or adults. The commonest underlying cardiac anomalies are valvar aortic stenosis, ventricular septal defect, and tetralogy of Fallot. Conversely, an ostium secundum atrial septal defect has never been described as the focus for endocarditis, and isolated pulmonary stenosis rarely, if ever. In Great Britain rheumatic heart disease is seldom found in children but in children from underdeveloped countries rheumatic mitral or aortic valve disease may provide the focus for bacterial endocarditis.

In approximately one-third of cases there is an identifiable precipitating factor such as dental extraction, cardiac surgery (or very rarely cardiac catheterization), infections such as osteomyelitis, or other surgical procedures.

Streptococcus viridans infection, usually from a source in the mouth, remains the most frequent organism causing subacute bacterial endocarditis although staphylococci, Gram negative bacteria, and other streptococci (in particular *Strep. faecalis*) are found. Acute bacterial endocarditis is extremely uncommon with congenital heart disease but can be caused by *Staphylococcus aureus*. It usually follows surgery and may complicate leukaemia or other serious illnesses with decreased resistance to infections. Candida endocarditis may be found as a superinfection during antibiotic treatment for bacterial endocarditis or after valve replacement. There is a particular risk from infected drip sites during prolonged intravenous therapy.

Clinical findings
Illness is usually present for three or more weeks before the diagnosis is made although a three-month history is not uncommon. Pyrexia, anaemia, and splenomegaly are found. A change in auscultatory findings such as might accompany the development of aortic regurgitation would strongly suggest the diagnosis. Focal neurological disturbances or generalized fits are found in infants while subarachnoid

haemorrhage occurs more in older children. Embolic phenomena occur especially to the lungs. Most of these features relate directly to the bacterial infection. Many of the other manifestations of bacterial endocarditis previously ascribed to microemboli could relate to immune complex phenomena. This applies in particular to petechiae, Osler's nodes (small painful nodules), splinter haemorrhages seen under the nails, arthralgia or arthritis affecting a single joint, retinal haemorrhages and exudates (Roth's spots), and haematuria.

Renal lesions
Microscopic haematuria is found in over 95 per cent of patients with infective endocarditis. The diffuse renal disease responsible for this is now thought to be part of the immune response rather than a microembolic phenomenon although frank major renal emboli can also occur. In older patients renal failure may supervene.

Laboratory diagnosis and treatment
Isolation of the infecting organism is mandatory for adequate antibiotic therapy. Transient suppression of fever by bacteriostatic antibiotics such as tetracyclines or by inadequate doses of bactericidal agents is dangerous as it may lead to delay in diagnosis while valve damage and the immune disease progress. A cavalier attitude to antibiotic therapy in patients at risk from bacterial endocarditis is to be deprecated.

For diagnosis, blood is taken with full antiseptic precautions and cultured aerobically and anaerobically. At least three blood samples are taken for culture before starting antibiotics. In patients referred to hospital already receiving blind therapy it may be necessary to discontinue antibiotics for up to 48 hours in order to obtain positive blood cultures. Therapy is dictated by the antibiotic sensitivities of the organisms isolated. Bactericidal drugs such as penicillin, cephalosporins or aminoglycosides (i.e. gentamycin) must be used rather than bacteriostatic agents such as tetracycline. Dosages are adjusted according to the concentrations of antibiotics in the blood. In children intravenous administration of drugs is kinder than multiple intramuscular injections. Oral therapy has been advocated by some but is not as reliable as parenteral therapy and is not used at the Brompton Hospital.

If the organism is sensitive, penicillin remains the drug of choice combined with a second bactericidal agent, e.g. streptomycin or gentamycin. The drugs are given as a bolus injection into the infusion tubing. The interval between injections depends on plasma levels. To monitor adequacy of therapy, blood is taken just prior to the next dose of antibiotic—for instance six hours after the last dose. Therapy is considered adequate if a fourfold dilution of this blood sample (trough level) is still bactericidal to the organism previously isolated. If this is not the case then either drug dosage is increased, the interval between injections decreased, or urinary excretion is slowed by agents such as probenecid. Therapy is traditionally continued for six weeks but patients must be carefully watched on cessation of therapy.

In contrast to adults an organism can almost always be isolated in children with infective endocarditis. Blood culture on Sabouraud's medium may be necessary for growth of *Candida* and may take ten days or longer.

Prophylaxis

Penicillin prophylaxis is advised for dental extractions in the majority of patients with congenital heart anomalies. Particular emphasis is given to this in patients with bicuspid aortic valves, ventricular septal defects, or mitral incompetence. In secundum atrial septal defects it is unnecessary. Penicillin (i.m. or a large oral dose) is administered one hour before the tooth is to be extracted and continued orally for three days. It is crucial not to commence therapy sooner as the oral flora will become penicillin resistant. In contrast to long term penicillin prophylaxis against rheumatic fever, long term penicillin therapy is contraindicated as prophylaxis to bacterial endocarditis. Rheumatic fever is prevented as the beta haemolytic streptococcus remains faithfully sensitive to penicillin whereas long term use of penicillin in congenital heart disease would merely ensure that bacterial endocarditis in an affected patient would be with penicillin resistant organisms.

Surgery

The wide range of antibiotics now available usually allow eradication of active infection. An important exception to this is if infection relates to foreign material in the heart such as an artificial valve, conduit, or patch. Under these circumstances the infected material may have to be removed surgically.

Another indication for surgery would be an acute deterioration in haemodynamic status following valve destruction. Thus emergency aortic valve replacement may be life-saving.

References

Hamer, J. and O'Grady, F. (1977). Infective endocarditis. In *Recent advances in cardiology* (ed. J. Hamer), pp. 447–471. Churchill Livingstone, Edinburgh.

Jawetz, E. (1962). Assay of antibacterial activity in serum; useful guide for antimicrobial therapy. *American Journal of Diseases of Children* **103**, 81.

Part III
General problems

44 Cardiovascular risk factors in infancy and childhood

Epidemiological studies performed in adults allow precise quantification of the risks of vascular disease. The Framingham study has shown that 'an efficient, practical set of variables for this purpose is a casual blood test for cholesterol and sugar, a blood pressure determination, an electrocardiogram, and a cigarette-smoking history. With this set of variables the risk of coronary heart disease can be estimated over a thirty-fold range and 10 per cent of the asymptomatic population identified, in whom 25 per cent of the coronary heart disease, 40 per cent of the occlusive peripheral arterial disease and 50 per cent of the stroke and congestive heart failure would evolve.' This is of particular importance because treatment of some risk factors, particularly hypertension in asymptomatic individuals, is known to decrease the subsequent incidence of vascular disease. There is considerable incentive to the identification of risk factors in children, since it would seem that intervention might be more successful at this age than in adults. For example, it is possible that a short period of treatment of hypertension in infancy might prevent the patient developing hypertension in later life, and might obviate the necessity for life-long antihypertensive therapy starting in middle age. Similarly, if there is a group of children particularly at risk from vascular disease and/or abnormalities of lipid metabolism, perhaps treatment by dietary manipulation should be started in childhood rather than in later life. The latter has so far been ineffective.

It has not yet proved possible to measure risk factors in infancy with the same precision as has been achieved in adults. The reasons for this are threefold. First, in adults risk factors can be measured in a retrospective manner and then confirmed in prospective studies. Secondly, prospective studies would have to be very long, the ideal prospective study of risk factors in infancy lasting at least 50 years. The final problem affecting the precision of risk factor measurement in children is the variability of the risk factors themselves. Thus, it is well known that blood pressure varies throughout the day in adults. It is not so well known that blood pressure varies in children also. Nonetheless, despite these difficulties and on the basis of adult studies it seems reasonable to suggest that the major potential risk factors which might be identified in infancy, childhood, and subsequent life are blood pressure, blood lipids, obesity, salt intake, smoking, and the contraceptive pill. These will each be considered in turn.

Blood pressure
Numerous prospective surveys have demonstrated the potency of hypertension in adults as a risk factor for cardiovascular disease. Until recently, it had not been possible to measure blood pressure accurately and non-invasively in infants. However, the Doppler technique has altered this as it is simple to use and is more accurate than previous methods such as flush, auscultation, or palpation, which can underestimate systolic blood pressure by as much as 45 mmHg. Although it is not yet possible in infancy to measure diastolic blood pressure with the same degree of accuracy this is of less significance since it gives no additional information as a risk factor, cardiovascular morbidity being more closely related to systolic blood pressure than to diastolic blood pressure.

It is known that there is considerable variability in blood pressure in children, not only within a 24-hour period but also when blood pressure is measured over a longer interval. This degree of variability has emphasized the necessity for longitudinal studies which will define precisely the relationship of blood pressure measurements made at one age to those made as the children grow older. Such a study is in progress at the Brompton Hospital. This is a population study of paediatric blood pressure starting in the neonatal period, the purpose being to establish the normal range of blood pressure in infants and young children.

The data thus far obtained from the Brompton study shows that the fiftieth percentile for systolic blood pressure rises rapidly from 75 mmHg at age four days to 95 mmHg at age six weeks (Fig. 44.1). It then remains stable until at least the age of one year. By comparing these findings with the data from the Miami, Muscatine, and Rochester studies pooled by the American Task Force for Blood Pressure Control, blood pressure appears to be stable from ages six weeks to six years (Fig. 44.1). The Brompton study has further shown that blood pressure measurements made as early as age four days are correlated with blood pressure measurements at age six weeks and it seems that the tendency to develop hypertension may be demonstrated in the neonatal period. More recent data has shown no correlation in blood

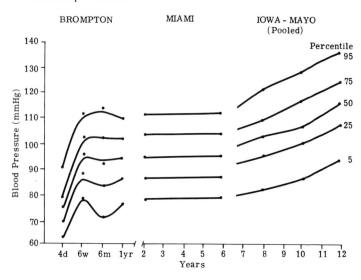

Fig. 44.1 Percentiles for blood pressure in the first 12 years of life. Data is taken from the Brompton Study for the first year, from the Miami Study the years 2 to 6 and pooled data from Iowa and Mayo studies are given for the years 7 to 12. It will be seen that blood pressure rises between 4 days and 6 weeks and then remains stable for the next 6 years.

pressures between aged six weeks and six months but the correlations reappear between the ages of six months and one year. At these ages, family relationships between children and mothers' blood pressure are also demonstrable. This and other data suggests that children do not develop blood pressures related to those that they would have in adult life until the age of at least six months. When comparing these findings with other studies it would appear that 'tracking' of blood pressure starts to be demonstrable in the first year of life but that the correlation in serial blood pressure measurements made at this age is weak. The significance of high blood pressure in childhood as a risk factor for subsequent adult cardiovascular disease is therefore weaker than that between blood pressure measured in adult life and the development of cardiovascular disease. Nonetheless, in one study it has been demonstrated that high blood pressure existing before the age of 25 years is associated with subsequent cardiovascular morbidity and mortality. It is probable that other studies will show a similar association if the follow-up period is sufficiently long.

Familial aggregation of blood pressure has also been demonstrated in the Brompton study from the age of six months but not at earlier ages. Thus, finding of high blood pressure in the parents may well point to the likelihood of development of hypertension in their offspring.

Blood lipids

Since the levels of various lipids in the blood have been shown to be related to cardiovascular morbidity and mortality, similar epidemiological studies to those already quoted for hypertension have been performed. Although several cross sectional studies are available there is less data on longitudinal correlations of blood lipid levels. If elevated blood lipid levels in childhood are to be considered risk factors their consistency must be demonstrated. Thus far, there is little evidence to show that 'tracking' of blood lipids appears. It is not yet clear whether serum lipid levels in adult life can be predicted from estimations made during infancy and childhood. The problem is compounded by the difficulty of defining normality of lipid levels in childhood. At birth, cholesterol levels are low (about 75 mg/dl) and are independent of variables such as maternal hyperlipidaemia, gestation, or ethnic origin. The level then rises within the first year of life to the level at which it remains for the rest of childhood. It has been suggested on the basis of epidemiological studies that 200 mg/dl should be the upper limit of normal for cholesterol in children. The data for serum triglyceride is even more difficult to obtain, for there are wide fluctuations related to the time of feeding. A fast of between eight and twelve hours is necessary to obtain reproducible values. Using these criteria, the suggested upper limit for children is 140 mg/dl. Children who have relatively modest increases in blood lipids are likely to have them in association with diet, or other secondary conditions such as diabetes mellitus. Large increases in blood lipids are likely to occur in the primary hyperlipoproteinaemias, particularly in the homozygous form. In these children, the serum cholesterol may be as great as 1000 mg/dl and they rarely live beyond adolescence. However, it is known that heterozygotes with primary hyperlipoproteinaemia have an increased risk of ischaemic heart disease compared to unaffected relatives.

Thus, levels of cholesterol persistently exceeding 250 mg/dl or of triglyceride exceeding 140 mg/dl are likely to be abnormal in children and probably indicate primary hyperlipoproteinaemia. Both hetero- and homozygotes have an unequivocally increased risk of vascular disease. More modest increases in the concentrations of blood lipids are much more common and their potencies as cardiovascular risk factors still remain unknown.

Obesity

Evidence from the Framingham studies suggests that much of the risk of obesity comes from association with other factors. It is correlated with raised blood pressure and cholesterol levels and with glucose intolerance. When these risks have been allowed for obesity has little additional contribution to make to the cardiovascular risk profile. Blood pressure is also correlated with weight in children. It is unlikely that neonatal obesity will be a very strong risk factor since approximately 70 per cent of babies overweight in the first year of life are of normal weight by age four to seven years.

Salt

Several epidemiological studies have linked a low salt diet with the absence of hypertension. However, others have found no relationship between blood pressure and sodium excretion.

In the Brompton study no relationship has been found between blood pressure between the ages of four days and one year and the method of feeding at age six weeks once allowance has been made for the increased weight of bottle-fed babies. Most bottle feeds, even if correctly mixed, have twice the sodium content of human milk. However, salt balance was not studied in the Brompton investigation and it is still possible that infants with higher blood pressures retain more sodium even though their total intake may be the same as those with lower blood pressures.

Smoking

There is clear evidence that smoking is a cardiovascular risk factor in adults. Smoking habits tend to be acquired early in life and are often familial. It would therefore seem desirable to dissuade 'at risk' families from smoking for the sake of their children's health. However, it remains to be seen whether this would be a significant additional reason for giving up the habit.

The contraceptive pill

It has been shown that taking the contraceptive pill in women under the age of 35 years interacts significantly with smoking, hypertension, diabetes, and Type II hyperlipoproteinaemia as risk factors for myocardial infarction. It is unlikely that taking the pill would add a risk in the absence of the above risk factors. However, on the above evidence, adolescents who are obese with elevated blood pressures should be counselled against using the contraceptive pill.

Conclusions and recommendations

As yet there are no hard data linking cardiovascular risk with risk factors present in infancy. Some potential risk factors such as smoking or taking the contraceptive pill are voluntarily accepted and susceptible children and adolescents should be actively discouraged from doing so. Other possible risk factors such as hypertension and blood lipid level are more related to the genetic make-up and the environment of the child. Therefore, more drastic steps are necessary to alter them. In these circumstances it would seem prudent to manipulate only the extreme examples until further evidence is forthcoming concerning the power of each individual risk factor.

References

Bewley, B. R. (1978). Smoking in childhood. *Postgraduate Medical Journal* **54**, 197.

de Swiet, M., Fancourt, R., and Peto, J. (1975). Systolic blood pressure variation during the first 6 days of life. *Clinical Science and Molecular Medicine* **49**, 557.

de Swiet, M., Fayers, P., and Shinebourne, E. A. (1976). Blood pressure survey in a population of newborn infants. *British Medical Journal* **2**, 9.

de Swiet, M. and Shinebourne, E. A. (1977). Blood pressure in infancy. *American Heart Journal* **94**, 399.

Lauer, R. M., Connor, W. E., Leaverton, P. E., Reiter, M. A., and Clarke, W. R. (1975). Coronary heart disease risk factors in schoolchildren: the Muscatine Study. *Journal of Pediatrics* **86**, 697.

Lloyd, J. K. (1976). Hyperlipoprotinaemia and atherosclerosis. In *Recent advances in paediatrics* (ed. D. Hull). Churchill Livingstone, Edinburgh.

Mann, J. I., Vessey, M. P., Thorogood, M., and Doll, R. (1975). Myocardial infarction in young women with special reference to oral contraceptive practice. *British Medical Journal* **2**, 241.

Rames, L. K., Clarke, W. R., Connor, W. E., Reiter, M. A., and Lauer, R. M. (1979). Normal blood pressures and the evaluation of sustained blood pressure elevation in childhood: the Muscatine Study. *Pediatrics.* In the press.

Report of the task force on blood pressure control in children (1977). *Pediatrics* **59** (Supplement—May 1977).

Strong, J. P. and McGill, A. C. (1969). The paediatric aspects of atherosclerosis. *Journal of Atherosclerosis Research* **9**, 215.

Zinner, S. H., Martin, L. F., Sacks, F., Rosner, B., and Kass, E. H. (1974). A longitudinal study of blood pressure in childhood. *American Journal of Epidemiology* **100**, 437.

Zinner, S. M., Margolius, H. S., Rosner, B., and Kass, E. H. (1979). Stability of blood pressure rank and urinary kallikrein concentration in childhood: an eight-year follow-up. *Circulation.* In the press.

45 Cardiac arrhythmias

The study of cardiac conduction abnormalities is one of the most neglected areas of paediatric cardiology. However, in recent years there has been growing appreciation of the importance of a clear understanding of their management, diagnosis, and treatment. From continuous ambulatory monitoring it is now clear that cardiac arrhythmias are a frequent occurrence both in children with congenital heart defects and in those without structural abnormalities of the heart. Furthermore the careful treatment of rhythm disturbances may be of vital importance, especially after cardiac surgery. In this chapter we have attempted to provide a basis for the understanding of the electrophysiological mechanisms responsible for the common arrhythmias so that a rational approach to diagnosis and treatment may be possible. In addition we discuss modern investigation and specific problems that occur in the paediatric age group. Those interested in the electrophysiological properties of conduction tissue are referred to the reviews of Nayler and Krikler (1975) and Rosen (1975).

Anatomy of the conduction system
The specialized conduction system of the heart consists of the sinus node, the atrioventricular node, the atrioventricular bundle (of His) and its branches, and the peripheral ventricular conduction fibres (Purkinje fibres). The sinus node, or pacemaker, is situated in the lateral part of the sulcus between the superior vena cava and the right atrium (Fig. 45.1). It has an inherently faster rate of discharge than any other structure in the heart, and its rate is controlled by an abundant autonomic nerve supply. Sinus node rate in the newborn is rapid and relatively unstable; that of the adult slower and more stable. Atrial depolarization produces the P-wave of the electrocardiogram. The atrioventricular node is located at the base of the atrial septum immediately adjacent to the central fibrous body. Its functions include the capacity to delay the sinus impulse during ventricular filling and to protect the ventricles when the atrial rate becomes excessive, and the ability to act as a secondary pacemaker in the event of failure of the sinus node. The impulse is conducted from sinus node to atrioventricular node through the atrial myocardium, the geometry of the right

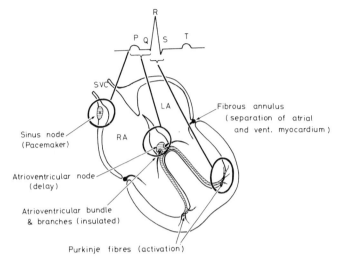

Fig. 45.1 Diagrammatic representation of the anatomy of the specialized conduction system and its relation to the fibrous annulus and the electrocardiogram. SVC = superior vena cava; RA = right atrium; LA = left atrium.

atrial chamber determining the presence of preferential pathways of activation. In the normal heart, the atrioventricular bundle is the only connexion between the atrial and ventricular myocardium, piercing the fibrous plane in the central fibrous body. Elsewhere the fibrous annulus and the tissue of the atrioventricular sulcus completely separate the atrial and ventricular musculatures (Fig. 45.1). The bundle branches pass from the atrioventricular bundle down each side of the muscular ventricular septum, separated from the muscle by a fibrous sheath, and pass into myocardium at the ventricular apices as the Purkinje fibres. Ventricular activation, which produces the QRS complex of the electrocardiogram, therefore proceeds from the apices towards the base of the heart.

Investigations

The ECG remains the mainstay of diagnosis and treatment in any patient with a history or arrhythmias. If patients with disorders of rhythm are not missed it is essential routinely to record an ECG in any infant with unexplained symptoms of syncope, convulsive episodes, dizziness, or dyspnoea.

The P–R interval of the electrocardiogram, recorded from the onset of the P-wave to the first deflection of the QRS complex, represents the time taken for the wave of depolarization to travel from the sinus node through the atrioventricular node to the ventricular myocardium. In children, both age and rate have to be considered in determining whether there is an abnormality of the P–R interval. In general, the P–R interval increases with age and is shorter at faster sinus rates. The P–R interval is normally short in infants and neonates, but this may also be seen when the pacemaker is not the sinus node, and with ventricular pre-excitation. Conversely, a prolonged P–R interval may reflect congenital or acquired delay in conduction, the latter being seen in rheumatic or other forms of myocarditis. The QRS duration is normally less than 0·08 s and is very little affected by heart rate or age. Prolongation of the QRS duration beyond 0·12 s usually indicates bundle branch disease; intermediate figures (0·09–0·11 s) may be normal or reflect incomplete bundle branch block.

It is only by careful inspection of each component of the electro-cardiogram that accurate diagnosis will be possible. The importance of recording all twelve leads whenever possible cannot be over-emphasized, particularly in the presence of tachycardia. It will then often be possible accurately to localize the site of the arrhythmia. Leads II and V_1 are most likely to provide the clearest definition of atrial activity (P-waves). It is important to study the configuration of the P-waves carefully and where possible comparison should be made with previous recordings during sinus rhythm. An alteration in the P-wave morphology suggests that the rhythm is not originating from the sinus node. Although the P-wave will usually precede the QRS complex it may be buried within or indeed follow it when the rhythm originates from a site distal to the sinus node. Fig. 45.3 shows a junctional tachycardia in which the P-waves are inverted and follow each QRS complex; the atria are activated retrogradely.

The intravenous use of drugs that act on specific areas of the myo-cardium has added a new dimension to the information that may be obtained from the standard ECG. It may be possible to demonstrate the presence of a concealed bypass tract by giving a drug that will selectively act on the atrioventricular node so that conduction via an accessory pathway will become evident on the surface ECG.

While an arrhythmia may not be present on the resting ECG, one can sometimes be provoked by exercise. The *exercise ECG* is now a standard tool in the diagnosis of tachycardias. Exercise is usually performed on a treadmill or bicycle though a simple step test may be all that is required. It is important that facilities for continuous monitoring and resuscitation are available. Provided careful precautions are taken, the investigation is extremely safe and may provide diagnostic information not otherwise available.

In recent years considerable advances have been made in *ambulatory monitoring* of the electrocardiogram. It is now possible to perform 24-hour monitoring in patients of any age including neonates. This has enormous advantages over single recordings. In the first instance paroxysmal arrhythmias not seen on resting or exercise studies may be identified when recordings are continued over 24 hours. Furthermore, information is provided about the number, severity, and duration of the attacks. All these factors are important when deciding about therapy. Also, it is now possible to assess, in the patient's home environment, the efficacy of treatment by objective measurements. Several systems are available though in essence they are all similar. Two electrodes are placed in a position where there is a good display of all the components of the ECG complex. Recordings are made on a small portable tape recorder which can be worn by the patient. Analysis is performed both by automated systems and by watching the ECG oscilloscope played through at 60 times normal speed.

Occasionally investigations using the surface electrocardiogram do not provide sufficient data to be able to define the mechanism of an arrhythmia in sufficient detail to permit optimal treatment. In these patients an *electrophysiological* investigation may be necessary. This invasive technique will allow a detailed study of the conduction system to be made and at the same time closely to observe the effect of treatment. The decision to investigate a patient in such a way must be made only after careful consideration. The significance of an arrhythmia and the prognostic implications can be determined. The most obvious example is atrial fibrillation in the Wolff–Parkinson–White syndrome, where ventricular fibrillation may occur if the bypass can conduct at rapid rates. Knowledge of the refractory period of the bypass will identify patients at special risk so that appropriate precautions can be taken.

For a detailed description of the procedures used to perform an electrophysiological study, the reader is referred to the reviews of Curry (1975) and Gillette *et al.* (1975). In essence, several bipolar pacing catheters are placed pervenously and placed high in the right atrium, opposite the His bundle, in the right ventricle and in the coronary sinus, the last to record and pace from the left atrium. The intracardiac conduction intervals (atrium–His, His–ventricle) are measured. It is then necessary to measure the ability of the atrioventricular node and any accessory pathway present to conduct stimuli presented at successively shorter intervals after the preceding beat. Pacing tests are performed to determine the ability of the sinus node to recover following repeated stimulation and to observe the effects of increasing heart rates on the atrioventricular node and any accessory pathway present. Suitably timed stimuli may induce reciprocating tachycardia, drug effects can then be assessed and, if necessary, such tachycardias can be terminated electrically.

At birth the speed of conduction from the sinus node to the atrioventricular node is similar to that in the adult. In contrast, conduction through the atrioventricular node and from the His bundle to the ventricles (HV) is quicker at birth, decreasing with age.

Mechanisms of arrhythmias

Before considering the mechanisms of bradycardia and tachycardia in detail, it is important to remember that conduction in an arrhythmia may continue either in a normal anterograde direction or some chambers may be activated retrogradely. Both the normal specialized atrioventricular conduction pathways and accessory pathways may conduct in either direction. Thus, in sinus rhythm, P-waves will be upright in

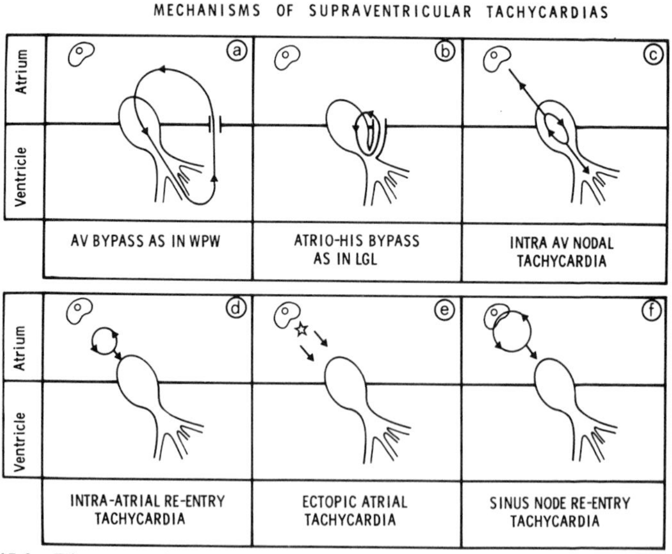

MECHANISMS OF SUPRAVENTRICULAR TACHYCARDIAS

Fig. 45.2 Diagrammatic representation of the various forms of focal and re-entry supraventricular tachycardia. (Reprinted with permission from Evans, T. R. (1979) Supraventricular tachycardia. *British Journal of Hospital Medicine.* WPW: Wolff–Parkinson–White syndrome; LGL: Lown–Ganong–Levine syndrome; AV: atrioventricular.

leads, II, III, and aVF. However, if the pacemaker is in the atrioventricular junction, the atria will be activated retrogradely with an inverted P-wave in these leads. Junctional rhythm with retrograde conduction via an accessory pathway will result in *tachycardia*. The electrophysiological mechanisms of both supraventricular and ventricular tachycardias is on the basis of either enhanced automaticity (localized focus) or a re-entry circuit (reciprocating tachycardia, circus movement) (Fig. 45.2). A localized focus of activity may occur anywhere in the conduction system. Re-entry circuits, on the other hand, occur when there is an additional conducting pathway or an area of abnormally slowed conduction, which will allow a circuit to be formed. The circuit may be totally confined to either the atria or the ventricles, may involve the atrioventricular junction, or may involve the atrioventricular node in one direction and an accessory atrioventricular pathway in the other. A minute circuit confined to atria or ventricles cannot be distinguished from a localized focus in many cases, nor, therapeutically, may there be much advantage in having this information.

The specific mechanisms that suddenly set off focal tachycardias are unknown, though ischaemia, electrolyte disturbance, and drug effects are important causes. A re-entry tachycardia is often set up when a critically timed extrasystole travels down one pathway and the return limb of the circuit allows conduction to occur retrogradely, thereby forming a reciprocating circuit (Fig. 45.3). The tachycardia will stop when another extrasystole renders part of the conducting system

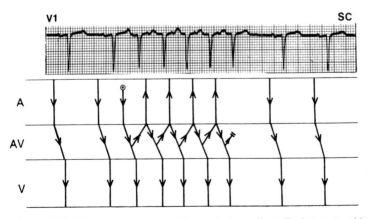

Fig. 45.3   ECG (VI) showing re-entry atrioventricular tachycardia that starts with an atrial extrasystole (third beat); after conduction to the ventricle, with P–R prolongation the atria are activated retrogradely (P′ follows the QRS).

refractory and the re-entry circuit is temporarily broken. In children, however, not every re-entry circuit is precipitated by an extrasystole and critical changes in the sinus rate may be responsible for almost continuous tachycardia (incessant tachycardia). Re-entry supraventricular tachycardia is best exemplified by the Wolff–Parkinson–White syndrome. In this condition there is an accessory pathway across the fibrous annulus, permitting abnormal conduction to occur between atria and ventricles. During sinus rhythm conduction from atria to ventricles usually occurs both via the normal conducting system (i.e. via the atrioventricular node) and via the accessory pathway. Indeed, only when there is conduction through the accessory pathway will it be possible to identify the condition on the surface ECG (short P–R interval, delta wave, prolongation of the QRS complex; Fig. 45.4).

CLASSIFICATION OF W-P-W

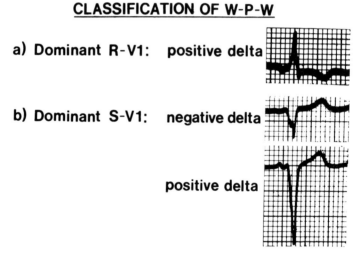

a) **Dominant R-V1:** positive delta

b) **Dominant S-V1:** negative delta

positive delta

Fig. 45.4 Classification of the Wolff–Parkinson–White (WPW) syndrome into type A (a) and type B (b) on surface ECG criteria. Note also short P–R interval and wide QRS with delta wave. (Reprinted with permission from Krikler, D. M. (1974). A fresh look at cardiac arrhythmias. *Lancet* **1**, 916.)

When an atrial extrasystole is conducted via the atrioventricular node to the ventricles the impulse may be conducted back to the atrium via the accessory pathway. Since anterograde conduction is through the atrioventricular node the QRS complex will be normal. In rare situations the circuit may operate in the reverse direction (antidromic) in which anterograde conduction is through the anomalous pathway and retrogradely back to the atrium via the atrioventricular node, the delta wave is exaggerated and constitutes the whole of the prolonged QRS complex. Understanding of this mechanism has important therapeutic implications. Drugs may be used which block conduction in either of the pathways, although the atrioventricular node is the easiest target for success. Alternatively, if these are unsuccessful, drugs that depress ectopic activity may suppress extrasystoles that might initiate tachycardia. In more refractory cases pacemakers which switch on automatically at the onset of tachycardia have been designed so as to induce a series of ectopic beats to interrupt the tachycardia. In the final resort, surgical ablation of the accessory pathway is available for intractable tachycardia or dangerous atrial fibrillation and may be needed in children. Disease of the sinus node, atrioventricular node or the His–Purkinje system, may all result in *bradycardia*. It is difficult in man to obtain information about sinus node disease. Even using intra-atrial catheter electrodes the action potential of the sinus node has not been recorded. To record a deflection from the sinus node would require that the electrode impales the specialized tissue itself, and this remains an unsolved problem. It is likely that primary generator failure of cells in the sinus node as well as entrance or exit block between the node and atrial cells are responsible for the sick sinus syndrome. Heart block, as generally understood, refers to conduction disturbance in the atrioventricular node and the His–Purkinje system. Either localized or generalized degenerative changes have been described.

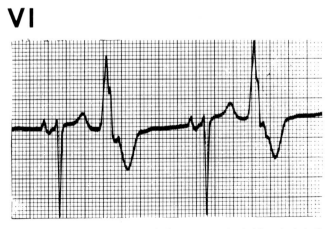

Fig. 45.5   ECG (VI) showing ventricular extrasystoles in bigeminal rhythm.

V4

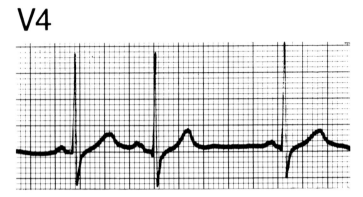

Fig. 45.6 ECG (V4) showing atrial extrasystole. Note the abnormally shaped P-wave preceding the ectopic beat (2nd beat) indicating that the impulse does not originate in the sinus node and the long P–R interval due to conduction delay in the AV node because the latter has not fully recovered after the preceding sinus activation.

Extrasystoles

Ventricular and supraventricular extrasystoles (Figs. 45.5, 45.6), although extremely common and benign, may constitute the triggering mechanism of both supraventricular and ventricular tachycardia. Re-entrant supraventricular and ventricular tachycardias are both initiated and terminated by extrasystoles occurring at a critical time. Focal tachycardias are a series of atrial or ventricular premature beats.

Supraventricular tachycardia

Though said to occur in approximately 1 in 25 000 children, the incidence is almost certainly greater since many cases must go unrecognized. Supraventricular tachycardia is usually paroxysmal but may be chronic. *Paroxysmal* supraventricular tachycardia is the most common variety and is found at any age though most commonly in the first year of life. In the infant and neonate the diagnosis may be made at routine examination and be unaccompanied by any associated symptoms. On the other hand, there may be severe haemodynamic disturbance, whether or not there are structural defects of the heart present, with clinical features of a low cardiac output associated with profound heart failure. Treatment should be urgent and immediate haemodynamic improvement occurs within minutes of restoring sinus rhythm. More usually symptoms and clinical signs lying between these two extremes are seen. In the older age group the symptoms and signs are initially less dramatic. The child may complain of a racing of the heart or the mother may notice a rapid heart rate; occasionally the child may feel faint. Ectopic beats preceding the tachycardia may be perceived but usually symptoms will start and stop suddenly and may last from a few minutes to several hours. At the end of the tachycardia, when sinus rhythm is restored, the heart rate may continue to be rapid (sinus tachycardia) for some minutes. In these circumstances a gradual slowing of the palpitations will be appreciated. Syncopal episodes or convulsions are less common but require urgent and energetic investigation and treatment. It is mandatory to record an ECG on any child with unexplained syncopal episodes or convulsions; ambulatory monitoring is necessary if the diagnosis is still uncertain. The ECG will characteristically show regular narrow QRS complexes preceded by an abnormally shaped P-wave. If a re-entry atrioventricular circuit is responsible for the arrhythmias, then subsequent retrograde atrial activation (P′) may be seen in addition, then usually meaning underlying preexcitation. If there is aberrant conduction the QRS complex will be wide and bizarre and it may be very difficult to differentiate this tachycardia from one that is ventricular in origin, though the former is favoured by finding the classical features of bundle branch block, right more often than left.

Either enhanced automaticity or re-entry may constitute the underlying mechanism of paroxysmal tachycardia. Myocardial cells in diseased atria (e.g. following myocarditis) may acquire pacemaking characteristics and digitalis toxicity, particularly in association with hypokalaemia, is a potent cause of enhanced focal myocardial activity. Re-entry circuits are, however, the most frequent basis for this arrhythmia. In addition to the Wolff–Parkinson–White syndrome other circuits involving the atrioventricular node such as atriofascicular and intranodal bypass tracts ('James fibres') have been described. When accessory pathways connect the atria and ventricles there will be a short P–R interval only when anterograde conduction is down the bypass; when conduction occurs exclusively through the atrioventricular node the presence of an accessory pathway cannot be established from the surface ECG. However, re-entry circuits connecting atria and ventricle can often be distinguished from focal tachycardias on the surface ECG. The most useful features are the presence of preexcitation on the resting ECG, and the use of carotid sinus massage. Pressure on the carotid sinus will not stop focal tachycardias but often slows the ventricular response by causing atrioventricular nodal block. In a re-entry tachycardia it will either stop the tachycardia or have no effect at all.

Chronic supraventricular tachycardia may present with short periods of sinus rhythm or as a chronic persistent tachycardia seldom if ever interrupted by sinus rhythm. This tachycardia is often resistant to conventional treatment. Digitalis may control the ventricular rate, and combined with quinidine, it may completely or partially inhibit re-entry. Amiodarone (not generally available at present in Great Britain) is most often effective.

Atrial flutter
This arrhythmia is important to recognize and can usually be distinguished from supraventricular tachycardia on the routine ECG if great care is taken (Fig. 45.7). Atrial flutter represents a continuous regular

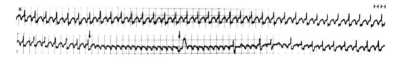

Fig. 45.7   ECG (lead II). Atrial flutter with 2:1 block (upper panel). The flutter waves become more obvious during carotid sinus massage (which was applied between the arrows) because of the induction of AV nodal block.

atrial tachycardia at a rate between 250 and 350 beats a minute. The ventricles respond usually in a regular fashion, usually in 2:1 to 4:1 ratio with ventricular rates of 70 to 350 beats a minute. It is important to examine all the 12 leads carefully for the presence of flutter waves particularly where there is a 2:1 atrioventricular relationship since these waves may be largely concealed in the QRS complex. By slowing the ventricular response with vagal manoeuvres the flutter waves may be rendered more easily visible (Fig. 45.7).

The haemodynamic effects of this arrhythmia depend largely on the ventricular rate and the presence or absence of co-existing heart disease. When associated with structural lesions of the heart (large atrial septal defect, Ebstein's disease, and 'congenitally corrected' transposition of the great arteries) the defects are often severe and usually there is severe congestive heart failure. The presence of underlying sinus node disease must be considered, and this may arise soon or long after surgery. While this is best recognized with Mustard's operation, it may also occur with repair of any malformation due to cannulation of the superior vena cava at the time of correction.

Atrial fibrillation

Here the atria are in continuous irregular motion at a rate of 400 or more times a minute. The ventricular response depends largely on atrioventricular nodal conduction but is always irregular and usually between 100 and 140 per minute. In the paediatric age group this rhythm is usually associated with severe structural heart lesions similar to those found with atrial flutter. The haemodynamic effects depend largely on the associated heart lesions but it is especially important in children with the Wolff–Parkinson–White (WPW) syndrome (see below). The possibility of underlying sinus node disease must be considered.

Ventricular tachycardia

This form of tachycardia is rare in infants and children. In approximately half of the patients no underlying cause will be identified. In the remainder, infection, injuries, cardiac tumours and drugs may be implicated, and about 20 per cent will have an underlying structural defect of the heart.

The diagnosis can usually be made from the surface ECG. The classical features are a rapid ventricular rate with bizarre QRS complexes and atrioventricular dissociation (Fig. 45.8). The first two of

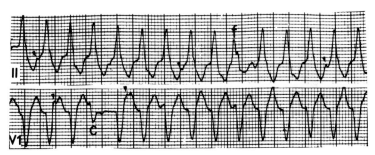

Fig. 45.8 ECG (lead II and VI) showing ventricular tachycardia with wide QRS complexes, AV dissociation (P-waves indicated by arrowheads), fusion beat (f), and capture (c) by sinus activation.

these features may, however, be seen during atrioventricular junctional tachycardia with aberrant conduction or pre-existing bundle branch block. Atrioventricular dissociation may not be seen if there is retrograde conduction to the atria when ventricular tachycardia cannot be easily differentiated from an arrhythmia originating in the atrioventricular junction. When there is atrioventricular dissociation, capture and fusion beats may be seen and their presence is diagnostic of ventricular tachycardia. Since this tachycardia is almost always associated with profound haemodynamic disturbance, a heart rate of between 180–220 beats a minute with a severely compromised circulation suggests a ventricular origin and in any case requires urgent intervention.

True ventricular tachycardia should be distinguished from '*torsade de pointes*'. This form consists of short bursts of activity with a changing QRS axis (Fig. 45.9). It may occur as a complication of heart block, the

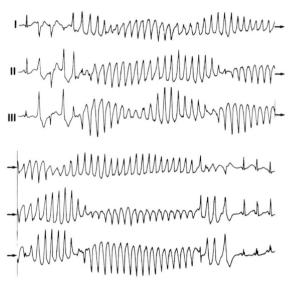

Fig. 45.9 ECG (3 simultaneous leads I, II, III) showing *torsade de pointes*. A burst of ventricular activity with a continually changing QRS axis.

prolonged QT interval syndrome (see below), hypokalaemia, and the administration of various drugs, particularly quinidine and phenothiazines. It must be distinguished from ventricular tachycardia due to intrinsic hypersensitivity to catecholamines when the attacks may be reproduced by exercise or the infusion of isoprenaline.

Sinus node disease

Only anatomical lesions should be considered as causing the sick sinus syndrome. Similar effects may be produced by drugs such as propanolol or digitalis or by alterations in the serum electrolytes, particularly hyperkalaemia, but these are transient and should not be considered as part of this syndrome. The sick sinus syndrome may occur in patients with organic heart disease such as cardiomyopathies and myocarditis, or develop after cardiac surgery. Sometimes there is no obvious organic heart disease, when it can occur as an inherited disorder (familial sinus node disease; prolonged QT interval syndrome, see below) or sporadically. The chronic form runs a varying course with periods of normal sinus node function alternating with abnormal behaviour. Symptoms include bradycardia and/or tachycardia, dizzy spells, convulsions, and syncope. Severe sinus bradycardia, intermittent or prolonged, must raise the suspicion of this condition. Paroxysmal atrial fibrillation without evident heart disease may be another clue. The sinus node may take several years to fail, whatever the underlying mechanism, and 5–10 years would not be unusual.

Heart block

All forms of heart block are rare in the paediatric age group in the absence of structural heart disease, intracardiac surgery, recognizable myocarditis (either non-specific or rheumatic), or drugs. Complete heart block, however, is seen as an isolated phenomenon. First and second degree heart block are not associated with symptoms. First degree block is manifest on the ECG as a prolonged P–R interval alone and most commonly accompanies digoxin therapy. Three forms of second-degree block are seen. Wenckebach (Mobitz type I) is characterized by a progressive lengthening of the P–R interval until an

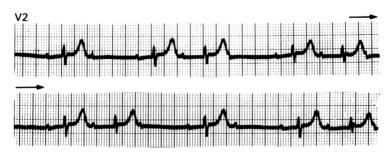

Fig. 45.10 ECG (V2) showing Wenckebach (Mobitz type I) second degree AV block. In this continuous recording the P–R interval prolongs progressively until the ventricular response is blocked.

anticipated ventricular response is blocked (Fig. 45.10). In Mobitz type II block the P–R interval is constant prior to the blocked ventricular response (Fig. 45.11). 2:1 AV block, where every second P-wave (sinus beat) captures the ventricles should be considered as a separate

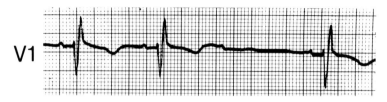

Fig. 45.11 ECG(V1) showing Mobitz type II second degree AV block. No QRS complex follows the third P-wave.

form of second degree heart block. The significance of these conduction disorders is that they may spontaneously progress to complete heart block. Until recently it was thought that Wenckebach heart block only rarely progressed to complete heart block, but studies have shown that up to 15 per cent of patients with complete heart block had displayed Wenckebach periodicity preceding the development of complete block. In complete heart block the atria beat more rapidly than the ventricles (Fig. 45.12). In most children congenital complete block

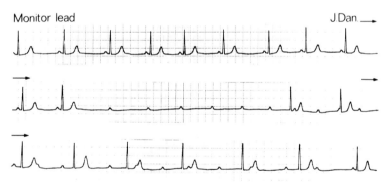

Fig. 45.12 ECG (ambulatory monitor lead) showing sinus rhythm (top panel) interrupted by ventricular asystole (middle panel) and followed by complete AV block.

is asymptomatic and compatible with longevity. The mortality in infancy and childhood, however, is estimated at not less than 5 per cent since Adams–Stokes attacks do occasionally occur and can result in death. It is often possible to identify the site of the block from the surface ECG; wide QRS if the block is low and narrow QRS complexes if it is high, though this is a broad generalization.

Pre-excitation syndromes

The WPW and related syndromes deserve special mention as they provide models for the understanding of re-entry circuits. Furthermore, the identification of these syndromes on the resting ECG may explain a history of paroxysmal tachycardia. The frequency of the WPW syndrome is estimated to be 1.5 in 1000. The usual basis of this syndrome is a lateral atrioventricular accessory pathway (bundle of Kent) which short circuits the atrioventricular node. This pathway provides a re-entry circuit on the basis of which supraventricular tachycardia may occur (see above). More sinister, though extremely rare in children, is the development of atrial fibrillation which may induce ventricular fibrillation.

The ECG in the WPW syndrome characteristically shows a short P–R interval, and widening of the QRS with a slurred initial deflection (delta wave) (Fig. 45.4). If there is a dominant R-wave in the right praecordial leads (type A) the bypass is left-sided, but if the QRS is predominantly negative (type B) the bypass is usually right-sided (Fig. 45.4). The typical complex is a fusion beat, caused by rapid conduction down the bypass which then merges with the normal cardiac impulse which traverses the atrioventricular node more slowly but is more rapidly conducted through the His–Purkinje system. The degree of conduction down either pathway may fluctuate with characteristic fusion beats or exclusive bypass or normal conduction.

There are several variations of the above syndrome, for example, conduction via an atrio-fascicular bypass tract (the Lown–Ganong–Levine syndrome) which is associated with a short PR interval with a normal QRS complex. Both must be distinguished from re-entry occurring within the atrioventricular node itself, but recognition of this may require specialized investigations.

Q–T prolongation syndrome

This syndrome is of particular importance as a cause of sudden death in children. In 1957 Jervell and Lange Nielsen first described an unusual syndrome consisting of congenital deafness, syncopal attacks, QT prolongation in sinus rhythm, ventricular arrhythmias, and sudden death. It is now thought that the syndrome may occur in no less than 1 per cent of severely deaf children; a similar problem may also occur in children with normal hearing. Characteristically the QT interval is grossly prolonged, in the absence of recognized secondary causes, e.g. hypokalaemia and drugs like quinidine, phenothiazines, or tricyclic antidepressants. Although the explanation of the prolonged QT interval is unclear, it is likely that the syncopal episodes are due to ventricular arrhythmias. The prolonged QT interval causes a prolongation of the vulnerable period, when a premature beat may set off the tachycardia. From the prognostic standpoint, syncopal episodes associated with a prolonged QT interval are potentially lethal and require treatment. There is evidence that the syncopal episodes may decrease in most children as they grow older. Treatment should therefore be aimed at depressing ectopic activity, propanolol being the drug of choice. It is unclear as to how long this should be continued but it would be wise if it were continued at least to the second decade. A similar but dominantly inherited disorder may occur in the absence of deafness (Romano–Ward Syndrome) and a *forme fruste* may be represented by a normal QT interval at rest that lengthens instead of shortening physiologically on effort.

Neonatal arrhythmias

Cardiac conduction abnormalities in this age group may go undiagnosed since often there are no obvious clinical symptoms. 24-hour (ambulatory) ECG monitoring will identify important cardiac arrhythmias in approximately 1–2 per cent of an unselected population. The importance of these latent abnormalities of conduction as the underlying mechanism of the *sudden infant death syndrome* remains conjectural.

Screening infants may identify those at risk. In the study of Southall and his colleagues a 10-second routine ECG strip was recorded in 2030 babies aged 6–9 days. Thirty-five were found to have arrhythmias or conduction disorders which may well have been considered benign. Ambulatory ECG monitoring performed on these infants showed episodes of supraventricular and ventricular tachycardia as well as heart block. Effective treatment may prove important in preventing sudden death in babies at risk.

Treatment

Understanding the type and mechanism of arrhythmia in an individual patient will facilitate a form of treatment that is physiologically sound.

The aim of *drug therapy* is to control the underlying mechanism, either enhanced automaticity or re-entry circuit. Broadly, drugs may be divided according to their effect on atrioventricular nodal conduction, His–Purkinje tissue, and the working myocardium. Thus digoxin, beta receptor antagonists, and verapamil all act by slowing atrioventricular nodal conduction. In contrast, membrane stabilizing drugs such as quinidine, procainamide, ajmaline, and disopyramide slow conduction through the His–Purkinje tissue and working myocardium. It is therefore possible to select a drug or combination that should provide the maximum antiarrhythmic activity for each individual patient. A patient with WPW syndrome may be treated with either an atrioventricular nodal blocking drug or one that works on an accessory pathway made up of working myocardium; alternatively, a combination of both types may be necessary. Where there is risk of atrial fibrillation with rapid conduction through the bypass, one should always select a drug that blocks conduction through the accessory pathway.

Both heart block and sinus node disease can be easily and simply treated using permanent *pacemaker systems*. These may be endocardial or epicardial though the latter is often preferable in children in that it is stable, will allow a redundant length of wire to be left for growth, and may be conveniently sited in the epigastrium.

Finally, in badly incapacitated patients with drug resistant re-entry tachycardias, *surgical interruption* of a bypass tract may be considered, though this is rarely necessary in children.

References

Curry, P. V. L. (1975). Fundamentals of arrhythmias: Modern methods of investigation. In *Cardiac arrhythmias: the modern electrophysiological approach* (ed. D. M. Krikler and J. F. Goodwin), W. B. Saunders, London. p. 39.

Gallagher, J. J., Gilbert, M., Svenson, R. H., Sealy, W. C., Kasell, J., and Wallace, A. G. (1975). Wolff–Parkinson–White syndrome: the problem, evaluation and surgical correction. *Circulation* **51**, 767.

Gillette, P. C., Reitman, M. J., Gutgesell, H. P., Vargo, T. A., Mullins, C. E., McNamara, D. G. (1975). Intracardiac electrography in children and young adults. *American Heart Journal* **89**, 36.

Gillette, P. C. (1976). The mechanisms of supraventricular tachycardia in children. *Circulation* **54**, 133.

Krikler, D., Coumel, Ph., Currey, P., and Oakley, C. (1977). Wolff–Parkinson–White syndrome type A observed by left bundle branch block. *European Journal of Cardiology* **5**, 49.

Krikler, D., Curry, P., Attuel, P., and Coumel, Ph. (1976). Incessant tachycardias in Wolff–Parkinson–White syndrome. I. Initiation without antecedent extrasystoles or PR lengthening, with reference to reciprocation after shortening of cycle length. *British Heart Journal* **38**, 885.

Nayler, W. G. and Krikler, D. M. (1975). Depolarization, repolarization and conduction. In *Cardiac arrhythmias: the modern electrophysiological approach* (ed. D. M. Krikler and J. F. Goodwin), p. 1. W. B. Saunders, London.

Rosen, M. R. (1975). Electrophysiology of the cardiac specialized conduction system. In *His bundle electrocardiography and clinical electrophysiology* (ed. O. S. Narula and F. A. Davis), p. 19. Davis, Philadelphia.

Southall, D. P., Arrowsmith, W. A., Oakley, J. R., McEnery, G., Anderson, R. H., and Shinebourne, E. A. (1979. Prolonged QT interval and cardiac arrhythmias in two neonates: sudden infant death syndrome in one case. *Archives of Disease in Childhood* **54**, 776.

Southall, D. P., Orrell, M. J., Talbot, J. F., Brinton, R. J., Vulliamy, D. G., Johnson, A. M., Keeton, B. R., Anderson, R. H., and Shinebourne, E. A (1977). Study of cardiac arrhythmias and other forms of conduction abnormalities in newborn infants. *British Medical Journal* **2**, 597.

Yabek, S. M., Svensson, R. E., and Tarmakani, J. M. (1977). Electrocardiographic recognition of sinus node dysfunction in children and young adults. *Circulation* **56**, 235.

Appendix PAEDIATRIC DRUG DOSES

Adrenalin Cardiac arrest and severe anaphylaxis
Neonate: 1 ml of 1/10 000 i.v.
Then 1 ml/year of 1/10 000 up to 10 ml ($\sim$ 0.1–0.2 ml/kg)
For status asthmaticus 0.01 ml/kg 1/1 000 s.c.
As an inotropic agent 1 mg/100 ml titrate against response starting with 2 microdrops/min. (0.06–0.6 μg/kg/min)

Arfonad (Trimetaphan camsylate) Ganglion blocker for post-op.
hypertension
250 mg in 250 ml titrate with blood pressure
Adult—starting dose is 60 drop/min

Aminophylline 4 mg/kg i.v.
Continuous infusion—0.7 mg/kg/h

Atropine Inhibits the vagus nerve
0.015 mg/kg i.m. or i.v.

Calcium gluconate (10 %) Cardiac arrest 0.1–0.2 ml/kg/dose i.v.
($\sim$ 1 ml/year of age – up to 10 ml)

Chloral hydrate 50 mg/kg orally hypnotic dose

Chlorothiazide 60–120 mg/kg/day orally in 3 doses

Chlorpromazine 1 mg/kg i.m.—pre-med.
0.25 mg i.v. for vasodilation (maximum 0.25 mg/kg)

Cardioversion 6 W. S/kg. Double, then quadruple immediately if no effect

Diazepam Drug of choice for convulsions
0.2 mg/kg/dose i.v. (slowly) ($\sim$ 1 mg/year of age) to a total of 10 mg.

Diazoxide 5 mg/kg in 30 s. Repeat in 1 h if necessary. Maximum of 4 doses in 24 h

Digoxin *Neonates: digitalization*
0.05 mg/kg/24 h in 3 doses i.m.

Neonates: maintenance
0.01 mg/kg/24 hrs in 2 doses orally or i.m.

1 month–2 years: digitalization
0.08 mg/kg/24 hrs in 3 doses orally
i.m. = 0.5 of oral dose
i.v. = 0.375 of oral dose

1 month–2 years: maintenance
0.01–0.02 mg/kg/24 h in 2 doses orally

>*2 years:* same as neonatal dosage
Given i.v. should be diluted with sterile H_2O to 1 ml and given over 15 min (to avoid heart block)

Disopyramide 2 mg/kg i.v. over 5 min. Then 0.4 mg/kg/h

Dopamine 2–10 μg/kg/min

Dobutamine 2–10μg/kg/min

Edrophonium 0.2 mg/kg i.v.

Ferrous sulphate 5 mg of elemental Fe/kg/day orally or 25 mg $FeSO_4$/kg/day orally

Frusemide 1 mg/kg/dose i.v., i.m. or orally (may double)

Glucagon 0.25–1 mg i.v.
May be given as continuous infusion (0.05 mg/kg)

Glucose and insulin For hyperkalaemia: 1 ml of D_{50}W/kg followed by 0.5 U/kg insulin i.v. Then maintenance fluid rate of D_{20}W for 2 h. Check response with Dextrostix every 15 min.

Heparin 100–150 i.u./kg/dose every 4–6 h as necessary, following clotting studies

Hydralazine 0.3–0.5 mg/kg/dose every 4–6 hours as necessary. Orally, i.m. or i.v. For post-op. hypertension in coarctation

Indomethacin 0.1 mg/kg orally. Repeat at 6 h and 24 h if necessary for ductal closure

Isoprenaline
Pump failure
Begin with 0.5–1 mg in 100 ml Dextrose. Infuse at 1 microdrops/min
In neonates concentration may need to be higher to avoid fluid overload (0.02–0.16 μg/kg/min)

Cardiac arrest
20 μg i.v. neonates 50 μg i.v. 1 year

Heart block/bradycardia
Drip with 1 mg/100 ml Dextrose. Start at 1 microdrop/min
Isoprel suppository (125 mg) 5 kg child =$\frac{1}{3}$ suppository
Saventrine tablet post-op. older child. Post operatively if pacemaker wires *in situ*, use them

Konakion (Vitamin K) 0.5–1.0 mg i.m. for newborns

Lignocaine 0.5–3 mg/kg/dose
Then continuous infusion of 0.5–3 mg/kg/h

Mannitol (20%) Oliguria (post-op.) 0.5 g/kg slow i.v.
Cerebellar tonsillar herniation 1–2 g/kg

Methyldopa *Oral:* Start with 10 mg/kg/day in 3 divided doses. Can increase to 50 mg/kg/day if no response. For chronic, not acute hypertension

For acute hypertension 2–4 mg/kg *i.v.* every 4–6 h. Can double the dose if no response in 4 h

Morphine 0.1–0.2 mg/kg i.v. or i.m.

Naloxone 0.01 mg/kg dose. For reversal of respiratory depression secondary to narcotics and diazepam. Can repeat as often as necessary

Omnopon 0.1–0.2 mg/kg

Pancuronium 0.1–0.25 mg/kg i.v. p.r.n. only if patient ventilated. Neonates 0.03–0.05 mg/kg)

Pethidine 1 mg/kg i.v. 2 mg/kg i.m. pre-med. dose

Phenobarbitone Oral: 3–6 mg/kg/day in 2 doses
   Acute treatment of convulsions—5 mg/kg i.v. Repeat in 15 min
   N.B. May cause respiratory arrest if combined with diazepam

Phentolamine 0.1 mg i.v. at 5 min intervals

Phenytoin Oral: 3–6 mg/kg/day in 2 doses
Acute treatment of convulsions: 5–10 mg/kg i.v. over 20 min
Same dose for severe digitalis toxicity
N.B. Do not give i.m.

Phenergan 1 mg/kg i.m. pre-med. dose
Sedation: 1–4 years 5 mg orally b.d./nocte 6–8 years 10 mg orally post-op b.d./nocte 8 years 20 mg orally b.d./nocte

Potassium chloride Post-op. dose 2 mmol/kg/day
   i.v. If K^+ is < 3.0 mmol/l give 1.5 g/500 ml fluid (20 mmol/500 ml)
   If K^+ is between 3.0–3.5 mmol/l give 1 g/500 ml (15 mmol/500 ml)

Procainamide 50 mg/kg/24 h orally in 4–6 doses

Practolol i.v.:
   0–8 months: 0.5 mg
   8–24 months: 1 mg
   2 y–6 y: 2 mg
   6 y–10 y: 3 mg
   10 y–14 y: 5 mg
   These may be repeated at 5 min to obtain the desired effect

Propranolol i.v.: 0.1–0.2 mg/kg/dose i.v. repeat in 2 min as necessary
   Oral: Arrhythmias 0.5–1.0 mg/kg/day orally divided every 6–8 h.

Prostaglandin E_1 or E_2
   1.5 mg in 500 ml Dextrose 0.05–0.10 μg/kg/min

Reserpine i.m. in post-op. coarctation 0.07 mg/kg i.m. repeat every 8–24 h.
   (Do not use in neonates and young infants)

Sodium bicarbonate Cardiac arrest: 1–3 mg/kg i.v. Repeat every 15 min
   p.r.n.

Salbutamol 0.15 mg/kg q.i.d. post-op.
  Infusion: 5 mg/100 ml 2–10 microdrops/min as necessary
  (0.2–1.0 μg/kg/min)

Spironolactone 1.5–3.0 mg/kg/day in 2 or 3 doses

Tolazoline 2 mg/kg i.v. then 1–2 mg/kg/h infusion

Vallergan For sedation 3 mg/kg orally. 4 mg/kg max.

Verapamil 0.05–0.2 mg/kg i.v.
  1–2 mg/kg 8 hrly orally (experience limited)

Warfarin 0.75 mg/kg orally. Loading dose divided over 48–72 hours. Then
  by prothrombin time

Index